SOLVED: *The Riddle of*
OSTEOPOROSIS

KEATS TITLES OF RELATED INTEREST

Solved: The Riddle of
Illness

• Stephen E. Langer,
M.D. and James F.
Scheer

The Calcium Plus
Workbook

• Evelyn P. Whitlock,
M.D.

Nutritional Influences on
Illness

• Melvyn R. Werbach,
M.D.

Dr. Wright's Guide to
Healing with
Nutrition

• Jonathan V. Wright,
M.D.

SOLVED: *The Riddle of* OSTEOPOROSIS

@@@@@@@@@@@@@@@@@@@@@@@@@@@@@@

SТЕРНЕN E. LANGER, M.D.
and JAMES F. SCHEER

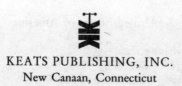

KEATS PUBLISHING, INC.
New Canaan, Connecticut

Solved: The Riddle of Osteoporosis is intended solely for informational and educational purposes, and not as medical advice. Please consult a medical or health professional if you have questions about your health.

SOLVED: THE RIDDLE OF OSTEOPOROSIS
Copyright © 1997 by Stephen E. Langer and James F. Scheer

Library of Congress Cataloging-in-Publication Data

Langer, Stephen E.
    Solved : the riddle of osteoporosis / Stephen Langer and James F. Scheer.
        p.   cm.
    Includes bibliographical references and index.
    ISBN 0-87983-785-3
    1. Osteoporosis—Popular works. I. Scheer, James F. II. Title.
    RC931.073L37   1997
    616.7'16—dc21   97-7975
                                                      CIP

Printed in the United States of America

Keats Publishing, Inc.
27 Pine Street (Box 876)
New Canaan, Connecticut 066840-0876

∾ CONTENTS ∾

∞ 1 ∞

THE ENEMY WORKS UNDERCOVER

Warning!

A lot of magazine and tabloid articles about osteoporosis—porous and weak bones—are dangerously incomplete, as full of holes as the degenerating bones they describe.

The purpose of this book is to offer you information as solid and strong as healthy bones to give you the complete yet simple story about how to prevent, stop or reverse osteoporosis.

Many people think, "My bones are O.K., so why concern myself with osteoporosis?"

Their problem is that the silent, subtle osteoporosis process may already be going on in their bones (no matter what their age) without their even realizing it.

Approximately 25 million Americans have osteoporosis, which results in 1.5 million fractures annually. Make no mistake, osteoporosis is a serious disease which can lead to brittle, easily broken, painful bones with one or more of these telltale symptoms: getting shorter, developing round shoulders or dowager's hump, sustaining fractures of the ankles, hips or spine—or, far worse, and, more excruciating—suffering a collapsed spine and even death.

IS IT HAPPENING TO YOU?

At first, bone degeneration is so slow and subtle that you're not even aware of it. You can't feel it in your bones.

Certain groups of people are more likely than others to develop osteoporosis. Osteoporosis affects more than three times as many women as men—those with a family history of osteoporosis, the small-boned, short, physically inactive women or—at the opposite pole—those who exercise so strenuously that their menstrual cycles are interrupted.

A particularly prone group is women who are tall and thin, are in the early or postmenopausal stage or have had their ovaries surgically removed.

Individuals of either sex are at equal risk if (1) they have neglected to take adequate calcium; (2) are undernourished; (3) regularly follow a high protein diet; (4) drink alcohol or coffee excessively; (5) are heavy smokers; (6) have a history of hyperthyroidism; (7) are on chronic steroid therapy; (8) are under incessant stress; (9) or have been bedridden for a long time.

CRUEL AND UNUSUAL PUNISHMENT FOR WOMEN

Eighty percent of the osteoporosis victims are women. Why is nature so seemingly unfair to women?

It's nothing personal. On an average, women are more small-boned than men. Their bones are thinner and less dense. So, from the start, they have less bone substance to lose before degeneration occurs.

Several studies reveal that women who get little or no exercise are decidedly more prone to develop osteoporosis than those who exercise regularly. This is also true of men, but to a lesser degree.

Too much long-sustained, grueling exercise, however, may be worse than too little physical activity. Women who habitually work out so hard that they stop menstruating lose bone minerals more readily than others and get an earlier start on osteoporosis.[1]

According to physiologist Christopher Cann, at the University of California in San Francisco, even continuous and extreme emotional stress can interrupt a woman's menstrual cycle and set off rapid bone destruction.[2]

Studies show that taking supplemental estrogen helps to prevent early bone demineralization. When premenopausal women have their ovaries surgically removed and stop secreting estrogen, their bodies respond as if they are in menopause, and their bones start losing substance, durability and strength, says Harry K. Genant, M.D., professor of radiology, medicine and orthopedics at the University of California in San Francisco.[3]

UNDERLYING CAUSES OF OSTEOPOROSIS

With osteoporosis, bones age faster than other parts of the body. We sometimes think of bones as solid objects which never change. That's incorrect. Like soft body tissues, bone cells are continuously recycled, losing old materials and developing new materials. This constant tearing down and building up— resorption and formation—affects both the tough outer bone surface and the spongy inner material.

Osteoporosis is a condition similar to a depleted savings account—more withdrawals from the bone bank than deposits. However, the money savings bank informs you in no uncertain terms about overdrafts. The body doesn't until the condition is extreme. And that's why you should be alert to certain warning signs.

EARLY WARNING

Degeneration of the jawbone—gum recession or a

partially visible tooth socket—is frequently an early warning that osteoporosis of the skeleton may soon occur or that it has already begun.

Cornell University's Lennart Krook, D.V.M., Ph.D. and Leo Litvak, M.D., Ph.D. and associates, conducted fascinating research, carefully examining jaws and bone structure of periodontal disease patients who had just died of other causes.[4]

In the process, they discovered the progression of loss of calcium: first from the jawbones—as indicated by shrunken jawbones—next from the ribs and vertebrae and, last, from arm and leg bones.

With shrinkage of the jawbone and tooth sockets, the supporting bone draws away from the teeth, loosening them while irritating and inflaming the gums, often to the point of bleeding. (The origin of the descriptive expression "long in the tooth" is the appearance of the elderly who are actually experiencing osteoporosis.)

Other revealing signs of possible osteoporosis are translucent skin on the back of the hands and, as researchers in Maine discovered, prematurely gray hair.[5]

Prematurely gray-haired patients and control subjects with normal hair color were recently examined by sophisticated bone measuring devices and their results compared. The patients who were prematurely gray showed far greater bone degeneration than the others who had normal hair color.

Why? The researchers concluded that certain genetic disorders can cause poor metabolism of vitamin D, which is necessary for the absorption of calcium. With insufficient calcium absorbed, the body, including hair, loses pigmentation. In addition, Australian scientists discovered a related fact—that a single gene for a vitamin D receptor also contributes to determining bone mass.

There are other revealing symptoms of osteoporosis, but, unfortunately, they may also be associated with other conditions—for instance, nightly foot and leg cramps and persistent low back pain.

Over and above the easily observable first symptoms of osteoporosis, self-diagnosis can become difficult. Diagnosis is best left to the experts. If you suspect a problem, you should have a thorough checkup by a bone specialist.

Once major osteoporosis symptoms are obvious, serious degeneration is already underway: the person can become shorter, a dowager's hump may begin to show and/or the patient may be stricken with arthritis-like pains in bones and joints.

Lifestyle changes, including proper nutrition, the addition of food supplements and exercise are advisable for everyone, but are especially important in slowing bone deterioration brought on by osteoporosis.

X-rays are not always the best diagnostic test for detecting osteoporosis. Bone degneration isn't shown by X-rays until about 30 percent of the bone is lost, and the condition is far advanced.

Your doctor, however, should order X-rays to detect fractures of the vertebrae and to confirm other fractures suggested by clinical evaluation. There are measurements by means of modern medical instrumentation that can show osteoporotic deterioration. If you know you have osteoporosis, this will motivate you to take proper measures to cope with it.

Bone scanners in many large medical centers can often detect the degree of deterioration. So can nuclear magnetic resonance (NMR), which does the job without exposing you to radiation.

Another way to detect osteoporosis is through certain lab tests which can also help to determine the progression of the disease. High urinary or blood concentrations of osteocalcin and bone-specific alkaline phosphatase help to identify patients who might respond best to therapy. These tests can also be used to determine response to therapy far earlier than the bone mass measurement techniques.

Don't play self-diagnosis Russian roulette with your bones! Be examined by a medical professional. What you don't know *can* hurt you.

BATTLE STRATEGY

A simple strategy can help you win the battle to prevent osteoporosis or help you to rejuvenate your bones. This involves a thorough look at your lifestyle and eating habits to discover which factors may be contributing to your bone deterioration.

One or more of the following could be the cause of bone loss: less-than-optimal nutrition, insufficient exposure to sunlight, physical inactivity and, in post-menopausal women, less than necessary amounts of estrogen and progesterone, female sex hormones. In a future chapter, we will show that a lack of estrogen may not be the only—or even the major—hormonal factor contributing to osteoporosis.

Without question today's living with its heavy accent on labor-saving devices—which make us less physically active—and eating nutrition-poor, processed food, and taking in polluted air, water and food contribute to prematurely deteriorating bones.

An unusual study in England reveals with the clarity of a lightning flash what factors contributed to solid and healthy bones of people who lived 150 to 200 years.[6] During the restoration of Christ Church Spitalfields in London's East End, a rare opportunity presented itself.

When scientists at the Wynn Institute for Metabolic Research heard that crypts of 87 women buried between 1729 and 1852 were opened, they seized the opportunity to compare bone density of the long-deceased women and today's women.

It was immediately obvious that the old bones were much stronger than contemporary ones. Bone loss was greater in modern postmenopausal women than in bones of the same age group of 200 years ago. Even today's younger women had more bone loss than many of their older counterparts of two centuries ago.

One of the Wynn Institute scientists, Belinda Lee, a specialist in bone disorders, declined to theorize as to all the causes of the differences. She stated, "We don't know why this is, but one factor may be the lower degree of physical activity in present-day women."

Certainly there was far more walking and physical activity in the horse-and-buggy days than there is today. Other expert opinions hold that two centuries ago, people ate organically-grown, nutrient-rich foods, where biblical crop rotation was practiced— in sharp contrast with today's individuals who eat many processed foods grown in worn-out, insecticide-poisoned, mineral-depleted soil.

Further, some authorities believe that environmental toxins also upset individual hormonal balance and interfere with proper metabolizing of food— consequently bringing about smaller and weaker bone structure.

∽ 2 ∽

JUNKY FOODS, JUNKY BONES

Poor nutrition with emphasis on junk foods creates a shortage of minerals, vitamins, protein and enzymes, some of which were never even suspected to have a relationship to building and maintaining strong bones.

Deficient or even marginal nutrition often speeds the onset of menopause, when bones lose their minerals two to three times faster than before. When one has little bone reserve, many symptoms of osteoporosis appear, including the more than 1.5 million annual fractures of hips, vertebrae, ankles and wrists in the United States each year.

Let's look at the most serious bone-destructive lifestyle habits, over and above submarginal nutrition: heavy smoking and excessive alcohol and coffee-drinking. Why does smoking contribute to osteoporosis? At first, it's hard to penetrate the smoke screen to get at the answer.

Although smoking is most noted for narrowing the arteries and capillaries, making more difficult the delivery of blood, oxygen and nutrients to our trillions of cells, there's more to the story. Oxygen deprivation and free radical assaults in smokers contribute to emphysema or lung cancer and to prematurely wrinkled skin. Even more important, oxygen-deprivation often leads to poor metabolism, so that smokers fail to get maximum values from food. Also, several researchers have discovered that menopause arrives earlier in smokers than in nonsmokers and, with it faster bone loss.

Many oxidants in cigarette smoke increase free radical production in the lungs. Therefore, lung tissue membranes become peroxidized. Unless there is sufficient vitamin E in the blood, these delicate living membranes literally become rancid and deteriorate, limiting lung capacity and ability to produce enough oxygen for metabolizing food. So there may be incomplete "combustion" of foods and consequent subnormal nutrition, contributing to osteoporosis and other degenerative conditions throughout the body.

The importance of vitamin E for protecting smokers from all forms of degeneration was demonstrated by a study in a Toronto hospital.[1] Cigarette smokers whose diets were supplemented with vitamin E

11

showed a lower degree of lipid peroxidation than those who were not supplemented. Free radical attacks increased once vitamin E supplementation was terminated.

BAD-GUY BEVERAGES

Large amounts of alcohol daily displace the intake of proper foods, contributing to malnourishment and bankrupting of available B-complex vitamins. Further, excessive drinking of alcohol damages the liver and kidneys, as well as the brain, and creates greater demands for certain minerals and vitamins. When these demands are not met, deterioration takes place throughout the body, including the bones.

Alcohol also limits the stomach's production of hydrochloric acid, necessary for the absorption of the various nutrients, calcium among them.[2] Additionally, alcohol interferes with magnesium absorption and contributes to its wholesale removal from the body. When magnesium is drawn into the urine and discharged, it takes precious calcium with it.

Among 96 chronic, male alcoholics, ages 24 to 62, 46 percent had osteoporosis.[3] Although osteoporosis is usually rare among people under the age of 40, 31 percent of the alcoholics were osteoporotic.

Caffeine, too, can undermine bones. We often take in more caffeine than we realize, because it is found, not only in coffee but in tea, cola beverages and some drugs and medicines. That great American institution, the Coffee Break, may, over a long period of time, contribute to bone breaks. Individuals who drink a lot of coffee daily have been found by researchers at Creighton University School of Medicine to be osteoporosis-prone.[4]

Sure enough, one or two cups a day won't hurt. However, three or more cups daily over the years may cause a slow loss of bone calcium. Another aspect of the Creighton study showed that people who drink a lot of coffee usually neglect drinking milk and eating other calcium-rich dairy products.

TROUBLE PERKING

Although few double-blind studies exist indicting caffeine, there is a great deal of clinical evidence that it can contribute to bone-depletion.

Consider this. Thirty-one women were asked to drink a cup of decaffeinated coffee at three different times daily. In two of the cups, three or six milligrams of caffeine were added. The amount of calcium excreted through the urine was much greater after the drinking of the caffeine-spiked decaf than after the plain decaf: 50 and 60 percent respectively, following the ingestion of the lower and higher amounts of caffeine.[5]

So much for the short range. Are the effects similar in long-range intakes of caffeine? Yes. Another study revealed similar results. One hundred and sixty-eight women, ages 35 to 45, demonstrated that calcium retained in the body steadily decreased with the increase of caffeine. Women who took in a great deal of caffeine daily retained less calcium than those who ingested little caffeine.[6]

Habitual coffee-drinkers—those who ingested about 50 percent more caffeine than the average— lost six milligrams of calcium daily, attributable to caffeine. If that doesn't seem like much, add up this deduction for 365 days a year over a lifespan.

SOFT DRINKS, HARD ON THE BONES

Threats to bones are not limited to caffeine-containing beverages. Soft drinks, with or without caffeine, can leach calcium from our bones, due to their high content of phosphoric acid. Several cans or bottles of soft drinks daily can add so much phosphorus to the diet that it may upset the calcium-phosphorus ratio and cause desperately needed calcium to be lost in the urine.[7]

One of my patients, a women in her mid-twenties whom I'll call Candace, had such a severe case of arthritis that she could hardly walk or move her arms to operate her computer.

"I'm desperate," she told me. "Three other doctors recommended that I continue to take aspirins.

I go through a bottle of them in a week. And that's got to stop, because my stomach's killing me."

I questioned her on all aspects of her lifestyle and found no clue to the arthritis, which should never have happened in someone so young. Finally, it all came out. She drank between six and 10 cans of cola drinks daily. Obviously the phosphoric acid in these drinks had tilted the calcium-phosphorus ratio in favor of phosphorus, which was draining calcium from her bones.

"You can clear up your arthritis and stop taking painkillers within a few weeks if you cut out the soft drinks entirely."

She did, and, sure enough, she was free of arthritis, pain and aspirins within that period. Candace's case demonstrated more dramatically than any other I have treated the importance of keeping the calcium-phosphorus ratio well in favor of calcium.

PROTEIN PROBLEMS

A protein intake above 50 grams daily for men and above 40 grams for women may also cause a significant loss of calcium. (Pregnant women and nursing mothers can use as much as 60 grams daily.) In order for calcium to be absorbed by the cells lining our intestines, we need some protein.[8]

This is a *must* for synthesizing the stomach enzymes that break down calcium for absorption into the bloodstream and for distribution to our trillions of cells. It is also necessary for making the collagen which cements calcium in the bones.[9]

"An excessive protein intake increases urinary loss of calcium . . . and might increase bone resorption [loss], predisposing an individual to osteoporosis," write Robert Garrison and Elizabeth Somer in *The Nutrition Desk Reference*. "This can be a problem, especially in the United States, where the typical American consumes two to three times the daily requirement of protein. In fact, some researchers speculate that it is excessive protein, not inadequate calcium intake, that predisposes a person to osteoporosis."[10]

SUGAR AND SALT: ENEMIES OF YOUR BONES

Refined sugars reduce one's ability to absorb calcium.[11] This is not true of lactose (milk sugar), however. Other sugars may also block the movement of calcium from the bloodstream into the bones.

As a matter of fact, a high sugar intake is not sweet to the bones. It increases the urinary discharge of essential bone minerals: calcium, magnesium, copper and zinc.

Some people make the mistake of shaking a blizzard of salt on everything. They eat a little food along with their salt. Excessive salt seems to hyperactivate the parathyroid glands, which speeds up the turnover of bone minerals, stealing calcium from the bones and flushing it out in the urine.

Consuming too much salt is especially harmful to those who ingest too little calcium or who absorb it poorly—the elderly, for example. "A Japanese study reported in the *International Journal of Vitamin and Nutrition Research* found that a high salt intake resulted in a loss of calcium in both men and women," writes Frank Murray in *The Big Family Guide to All the Minerals.* "Thus, said the researchers at the National Institute of Health and Nutrition in Tokyo, high sodium diets may increase the risk of bone loss."[12]

PHYTIC ACID: A SERIOUS PROBLEM?

Over and above seasonings which can contribute to osteoporosis is a product in natural foods that does the same thing: phytic acid, found in whole grains, soybeans and peanuts.

Phytic acid combines with calcium, making it indigestible. The body then treats this duo as a waste product and throws it off.[13]

However, there is some offsetting news about phytic acid. Biochemist R. Ballentine writes that if we are on a nutrition-rich diet—which includes ingesting enough calcium—the phytic acid will do little harm to us.[14]

Nutrition authority L.D. McBean states that the intestinal tract may contain an enzyme which splits phytic acid. Additionally, an adequate intake of vitamin D will probably eliminate any problems from phytic acid.[15]

McBean offers a tip on bread baking which may also alleviate possible damage from phytic acid. When bread dough is leavened—raised with yeast— an enzyme destroys the phytic acid. This protective process does not work when baking powder is used instead of yeast.

Like phytic acid, oxalic acid in foods such as beet tops, chocolate, rhubarb and spinach captures calcium and draws it out of the body.[16]

PHOSPHORUS: KEEP THE RATIO RIGHT!

As mentioned earlier, in the case study of Candace, phosphorus, essential to good bones, removes calcium from the blood and bones when ingested excessively. Eggs, meats and organ meats are especially rich in this mineral. Various studies show that the intake of dietary phosphorus should never be equal to that of calcium. Rather, the ratio should not be more than one unit of phosphorus to two or two and a half of calcium.

A number of over-the-counter medicines highly touted in advertising are calcium antagonists: antacids, aspirin and mineral oil. New research indicates that most stomach upset is caused by too little digestive acids instead of too much.[17]

Antacids, of course, inactivate hydrochloric acid and, for those already lacking this acid, further aggravate stomach problems and, specifically, intercept the digestion and absorption of calcium, causing it to be eliminated.[18]

Aspirin and mineral oil also cause calcium loss. What's that? I can hear you object: Nobody takes in mineral oil! Maybe so, maybe not. Mineral oil is used in many cosmetic products and enters the body through pores of the skin. Abandoned long ago by knowledgeable people as a laxative, mineral oil prevents calcium and phosphorus from reaching the bones and, at the same time, steals valuable vitamin D, absolutely essential for absorption of calcium and phosphorus.[19]

∾ 3 ∾

GET OUT IN THE SUN!

You don't necessarily absorb sufficient calcium, even on a calcium-rich diet, if you don't get in enough sunshine to assure yourself adequate vitamin D. (Of course, you *can* take in enough vitamin D with fish liver oils or a vitamin D supplement.)

Several experiments show that daily exposure to about 15 minutes of sunlight or skyshine in subtropical or tropical zones throughout the year helps to create solid bones. Sunlight's ultraviolet rays interact with ergosterol, a form of alcohol in the skin, and by means of a complicated process, create vitamin D. People in temperate zones who spend time outdoors may get enough sun exposure in summertime. However, in other seasons they may need supplementation of this vitamin.

People who live farther from the tropics, where the sunshine is infrequent or weak, get little vitamin D benefit from the sun. Then, too, residents of smoggy metropolitan areas in any zone may be partially insulated against sunshine.

THE SUN AND YOU

In addition, individuals who live or work indoors, or are on the swing or night shift, sleeping during much of the day, frequently lack vitamin D. Therefore, they may need a vitamin D supplement.

Round shoulders and backs, as well as dowager's hump, are common in northern areas where sunlight is weak—particularly in northern Scotland—and even in hot and sunny regions of the Middle East for women who, for religious reasons, keep their heads and bodies well covered.

Late in the year, when the sun goes south for the winter, we in the northern hemisphere could benefit by going along with it—just for the health of it, because brief daily exposure to sunlight is one of the best and lowest-cost insurance policies for keeping us and our bones fit.

Many years ago, scientists observed that people in the tropics and subtropics usually had well-formed and sound bones and teeth, thanks to sun-activated vitamin D. But they were puzzled as to why most heavily-clad Eskimos in the far north, where the sun's power is weak, seemed to have just as strong teeth and bones. Eventually, they learned that Eskimos virtually ate their sunlight, deriving vitamin D from fish and fish liver oils.

THE ANCIENTS WERE SAVVY ABOUT THE SUN

Even though they didn't understand the science underlying health benefits from the sun, the ancient Egyptians knew that exposure to sunlight prevented rickets, the bending and distortion of children's limbs, softened bones, poor teeth, profuse sweating and extreme tenderness of the skin to touch. Therefore, they practiced regular and brief sunbathing.[1]

Archaelogists have found stone plates bearing the likenesses of Pharaoh Akhenaton and his wife Nefertiti giving their rachitic children sunbaths. Egyptians were noted down through history for having at least brief exposure to sunlight each day.

In the book *Sunlight and Health* Michael J. Lillyquist details parts of an illuminating article about the studies by E.V. Wilcox, M.D. of Herodotus's writings in 450 B.C.[2]

Touring a battlefield on which Persians and Egyptian soldiers had warred 75 years previously, Herodotus examined skeletons of fallen soldiers and made a remarkable observation. Skull bones of Persians were so thin and fragile that a pebble thrown at them would easily break through them.

However, the skulls of Egyptians were invariably so thick and strong that Herodotus could hardly break them with a stone. Dr. Wilcox elaborates the Herodotus findings in these words:

". . . from childhood, the Egytians shave their heads, and the bone is thickened by exposure to the sun. For the same reason, they do not become bald. Of all races of men, bald heads are rarest among the Egyptians. Such then is the reason for their strong skulls. And the reason why the Persians have weak skulls is that they cover their heads all their lives with felt hoods . . ."

Wealthy Greeks and Romans of 2,000 years ago had solariums in their homes, encouraging sunbathing for better health. Some individuals sunbathed on the roofs of their homes.

Actually, the fact that sunshine prevents rickets in children and soft, flexible bones in adults (now known as osteomalacia) was a scientific fact of life way back in 1796. In that year, the German University of Göttingen honored a researcher named J.C. Ebermeier with a special prize for revealing the effects of sunlight on the human body.[3] Ebermeier was among the first scientists to realize that rickets occurred in low-lying, dark and damp areas, rather than dry and light areas.

BOWLEGS, KNOCK-KNEES AND VITAMIN D DEFICIENCY

In those days, long before the worldwide web existed, word of discoveries traveled with glacial speed. Further, then, as now, there was resistance by the establishment against a finding that disturbed the status quo. The not-invented-here factor existed then, but didn't yet have a name.

As far back in English history as the 1600s, the degenerative disease rickets—bowlegs and knock-knees are typical signs—was so common that people and doctors accepted it as a normal condition—even King Charles I's own physician![4]

His explanation? The bones and joints hadn't as yet knitted together properly. Slowly the condition became acknowledged as a disorder of unknown origin.

A little more than a century ago, London, England was referred to as "the rickets capital of the world."[5] No other major city had as many cases per capita. Fairly far north, London, with its pall of coal smoke, row after row of tall buildings and narrow streets, where the sun could hardly enter, was the ideal environment for rickets to flourish.

Homes of the poor were sun-deprived, because there was a heavy tax on the number of windows in dwellings, and the people were forced to choose food over sun exposure. This tax was repealed in 1851.[6]

THE SUN AND CLASS DISTINCTIONS

Royalty and upper classes in 19th-century England purposely deprived themselves of sunlight and, unwittingly, contributed to poor bones and teeth. Particularly, the women intentionally stayed pale because such skin was regarded attractive and, further, it showed that they were of high social standing, a part of the leisure class, distinguished from the sunburned and sun-browned workers in farms and field.

However, with the Industrial Revolution, laborers in factories, too, had a pallor—unhealthy at that. Then a lightly tanned skin in winter became a status symbol of upper class society, indicating persons with the means for traveling south in winter.

Another historical reference demonstrates clearly the value of sunlight in promoting solid bones and teeth and good health. The rapid and unexplained physical decline of miners in England caught the attention of the government. Healthy individuals who began working in the claustrophobic confinement and darkness of coal mines often become pale and sick within months.

FINDING CAUSES

The Royal Commission investigated why so many long-time miners had crooked, distorted limbs and an eventual drop in energy, being so debilitated that some could no longer work.[7] The Commission found many illnesses: dermatitis, rheumatism, aching joints, anxiety, tremors and loss of balance, as well as tuberculosis. Osteoporosis was not as yet identified.

In England early in the 1800s, cod liver oil became a folk medicine with the reputation for preventing or stopping the progress of rickets. In 1919, Sir Edward Mellanby proved that a substance in cod liver oil was responsible for its curative effects—a substance later known as vitamin D.

Even early in the 20th century, scientific investigators were not sure that exposure to sunlight could prevent rickets. Then a researcher in Switzerland observed that children living in deep valleys where little sunlight could penetrate often had rickets. Children living on nearby sunny mountains didn't.

An explosion of interest in the healing power of the sun occurred in the United States in 1914 when an article in the popular *Literary Digest* revealed many benefits from sun exposure.[8] People started building homes with sun rooms, whose windows could be open to permit full value from ultraviolet rays. An old Italian proverb offers this truism about a home: "If the sunlight cannot enter, the doctor soon will."

Four things separate us from the sun and its benefits: clouds, smog, clothes and window glass. It is up to us to prevent the separation from becoming a total divorce. We can't do a thing about clouds. We can do a little to prevent smog. However, we can do a lot about the kinds of clothing we wear and keeping windows open, if we can't get outside.

W.O. Loomis, M.D., professor of biochemistry at Brandeis University, considers the deficiency disease rickets to be the first air pollution disorder, because air pollution in many cities reduces the amount of sunlight that can get through.[9]

In a survey, Dr. Loomis discloses that rickets is far more prevalent in northern regions of the world than in the southern.[10] Eighty percent of the children between two and three years of age in New Haven, Connecticut showed clinical evidence of rickets. Only 12 percent of children in Puerto Rico in that age bracket show such signs.

In his best-selling *Mega-Nutrients*, H.L. Newbold, a prominent New York City medical doctor, offers the gist of a presentation at a meeting on how light influences the body.[11] This was attended by scientists from 87 universities and major industries and goes far beyond vitamin D.

Dr. Newbold tells of a film showing hyperactive children in a routine hour in their classroom. They were incapable of paying attention. They twisted like contortionists in their seats, kicked at one another, crawled over and under their desks, or ran around the classroom.

"These children were enough to make a saint hit them over the head with a Bible," he writes. Then classroom fluorescent lighting tubes were replaced by full-spectrum lighting tubes—man's imitation of the sun's full range of rays.

After several months of daily exposure to full-spectrum lighting, the second half of the film was completed, showing the children no longer hyperactive, but calmed down, attentive to teaching and interacting with one another in a civilized way.

Dr. Newbold paraphrases a statement by Professor Richard J. Wurtman of the Massachusetts Institute of Technology, as noted for his experiments with interactions of light and people as for those involving nutrition and emotions and the brain.

"Dr. Wurtman declares flatly that light is the most important environmental input, after food, in controlling bodily functions."

Then Newbold shows an influence of light beyond the considerable contribution of vitamin D— on the pineal gland which secretes the hormone melatonin, which circulates in the bloodstream and can easily pass through the blood-brain barrier.

"Once inside the brain, melatonin apparently causes an increase of serotonin—one of a group of substances known as neurotransmitters," writes Dr. Newbold. "A neurotransmitter is a chemical that allows one nerve cell to stimulate another nerve cell . . . It is hardly possible to overemphasize the role played by these neurotransmitters in influencing mood and behavior."

Granted that light from the sun and from other sources is far more influential on our body and behavior than many of us believe. However, it is well to remember that our friend the sun can become our enemy if we are overexposed to it. Research reveals to doctors and their patients that overexposure to sun can cause skin cancers and damage to the eyes—particularly cataracts. Today, authorities hold that, with the diminishing of the ozone layer, excessive sunlight is a definite threat to those who frequently sun themselves for long periods—especially individuals with a fair skin.

FULL-SPECTRUM LIGHTS FOR HEALTH

When Edison invented the first electric light, people were happy just to have clean and steady illumination to replace sputtering and dripping candles and lamps fueled by smelly natural gas or kerosene.

Sunlamps are popular in some homes. For the past several decades, some manufacturers have designed and marketed full-spectrum lights, in an effort to include the entire range of the sun's illumination.

Two societies were created for the express purpose of providing the health benefits of full-spectrum lights: the American Society for Photobiology and the Environmental Health and Light Research Institute. Essentially, they are trying to create sunshine inside buildings.

An important contribution to knowledge and

health was made by an experiment of MIT's Professor Wurtman, in a home for the senior retired.

As described in Dr. Newbold's *Mega-Nutrients*: "The home's elderly residents were divided into two groups. One group was exposed to full-spectrum light in its day-to-day activities; the other group was not. At the end of the experimental period, the patients in the group exposed to full-spectrum light stimulation showed a marked increase in the absorption of calcium from their food intake."[14]

Dr. Newbold likens a 40-hour week's exposure to full-spectrum lighting to staying outdoors at noon for 31 minutes once a week in summer sunshine.

More and more, full-spectrum lighting is appearing in offices and industrial plants of progressive companies and in some nursing homes and hospitals. The Navy is now using it in submarines, because benefits go beyond building better bones. Of submarine use, Dr. Newbold writes: "This stimulation has not only been found helpful in preventing infections, but also in maintaining the men's health under the stressful, confined conditions of their tours of duty."

Fortunately, full-spectrum lighting is not much more expensive than conventional lighting, for home, office or industrial use, and is available in electrical supply houses and in some health food stores.

∽ 4 ∽

BEAT OSTEOPOROSIS
WITH SUPERNUTRITION

One of the greatest enemies of your nutrition program and your bones is physical inactivity. If this
sounds contradictory, it really isn't. If you're laid
up in bed, confined to a wheel chair or rendered
motionless in a cast, you're going to be robbed of
key bone minerals. "Use it or lose it" seems to be
what Mom Nature is telling us.

Look what happens to astronauts when confined
and limited in activity within a space vehicle: they
lose an average of 200 mg of calcium daily.[1]

Various experiments reveal that healthy volunteers
held rigid in casts from waist to ankles continuously
lose vast amounts of calcium, phosphorus and magnesium—all critical bone constituents.

People confined to bed for long periods usually

31

develop what is called "immobilization osteoporosis," due to insufficient use of muscles and bones and exposure to the sun. What's the best way to stop mineral loss from this cause? Sure, mineral supplementation helps. So do in-bed exercises. However, research shows that just standing for a few hours daily slows or even stops excessive mineral escape.[2] This fact disclosed to researchers that the force of gravity is important to calcium retention. Physical activity is almost as essential to healthy bones as supernutrition.

GOOD NEWS AND BAD NEWS

Many studies reveal that not exercising causes flesh to become flabby and bones to demineralize rapidly. This was demonstrated by an experiment at Teijin Institute for Biomedical Research in Hino, Japan.[3] Rear limbs of rats were held motionless in a plaster cast. Some of the animals were fed vitamin D for six weeks and then compared with the control group. The rats held motionless and without vitamin D showed devastating bone loss.

Rats on vitamin D showed a gain of bone weight and more calcium and phosphorus, leading researchers to conclude that the supplementation of vitamin D "diminished the effect of immobilization in the development of osteoporosis without any side effects." This is worthy of note by the bedridden and those who care for them.

Researchers in the Department of Oral Medicine, School of Dentistry at the University of California in San Francisco, gave healthy men kept in bed for experimental purposes 10 milligrams of fluoride in divided doses each day. However, this measure failed to afford the desired protection.[4]

CALCIUM CRISIS

Well-founded scientific observation tells us that 99 percent of your calcium is in your bones and teeth. Just one percent of it circulates in your blood or remains in body fluids between your cells. However, this one percent must be maintained for wellness—actually, for survival.

Why is this a must? Because calcium is needed in higher-priority parts of the body. It is essential for reproduction and growth, for contributing to the synthesizing of hormones, for helping (along with other nutrients) to keep cell membranes flexible so that nutrients can come in and waste matter go out.

The greatest basic need for calcium is to help the heart muscle to contract and maintain a steady rhythm. Laboratory animals deprived of calcium showed an enlarged heart which fluttered, rather than beat, a condition called fibrillation.

CALCIUM'S OTHER ROLES

Although not as great a contributor as vitamin K to blood clotting, calcium has a role in this function. Patients with a severe shortage of calcium in their blood could bleed to death. Subnormal calcium levels can also contribute to constipation, because intestinal muscles are often too weak for the contractions that are necessary for bowel movements.

Calcium is essential for the nervous system. With a marked deficiency of this mineral, nerve impulses cannot be transmitted properly, and the nervous system becomes overly excitable. Nerve fibers "fire" when they're not supposed to, causing involuntary muscle twitching, spasms, cramps and convulsions. Extreme cases such as this—called tetany—can even kill.

When the diet is low in calcium or other key nutrients, when there is little sun exposure and physical exercise, the body compensates by drawing calcium from bone structures.

Why delay protective measures until osteoporosis shows its ravages in the mouth, the hips, backbone or ankles and wrists?

The intake of additional calcium often helps. Milk, yogurt and cheese or fresh green vegetables can supply this mineral and many other nutrients needed to win the battle. However, before creating a special list of foods for this purpose, it would be best to note what mineral and vitamin deficiencies invite osteoporosis. Let's start with the all-important mineral calcium.

Abundant studies show with glaring clarity that calcium is a good starting point for defeating osteoporosis—at any age. However, the research of Dr. Charles H. Chesnut, professor of medicine and radiology at the University of Washington, reveals that the best way to cure osteoporosis is to prevent it with a supernutritious diet during the teen years when the skeleton develops its greatest bone density.[5]

That's not good news for those of us who graduated from the teens eons ago. The amount of calcium taken in during these years determines the solidity and sturdiness or the porosity and fragility of the bones forty years later.

An Authority's Regimen

Thirty-one 14 year-old girls interviewed by Chesnut were taking from 200 to 1,600 milligrams of calcium daily from dairy products or from a supplement—with an average of almost 1,000 mg.

Twenty-five percent of the girls ingesting less than 800 mg daily were calcium-deficient. One glass of milk offers about 250 mg of calcium. A quart of milk—four glasses—provides about 1,000 mg.

Something unusual occurred in the girls whose daily intake of calcium in foods and supplements was in the highest range, 1,500 to 1,600 mg. Chesnut found that they absorbed more calcium and retained more in their bones than girls on lower intakes.

An in-depth study of calcium supplementation and bone mineral density in adolescent girls tells us that rapid increases in bone density of children and young adults occur during puberty in both sexes, and peak bone density is achieved near the age of 20 years.[6]

Ninety-four preteen girls and teens served as volunteers. Their bone mineral density and bone mineral content of the lumbar spine and total body were measured by dual-energy X-ray absorptiometry and calcium excretion from 24-hour urine specimens.

Calcium intake from daily foods averaged 960 mg for the entire study group. The supplemented group received 354 additional mg of calcium daily. The placebo group received only look-alike supplements. Compared with the placebo takers, the calcium supplementers had greater increases in lumbar spine density by approximately three percent: 18.7 percent vs. 15.8 percent.

Conclusions of the study, as stated by the authors:

Increasing daily calcium intake from 80 percent of the recommended daily allowance to 110 percent via supplementation with calcium citrate malate resulted is significant increases in total body and spinal bone density in adolescent girls. The increase of 24 grams of bone gain per year among the supplemented group translates to an additional 1.3 percent in skeletal mass during adolescent growth, which may provide protection against future osteoporotic fracture.

COOPERATE WITH YOUR CALCIUM!

Dr. Robert P. Heaney of Creighton Medical School in Omaha, a calcium authority, considers the RDA of 800 mg for calcium low, and recommends 1,500 mg per day. And a daily intake of 2,500 mg of calcium would help most women without harming them, he claims.[7]

For milk-intolerant individuals, Heaney suggests alternative calcium-rich foods: salmon, sardines— soft, edible bones remain in canned versions—sesame seeds, soybeans, almonds, brazil nuts, pistachios and sunflower seeds, along with leafy greens.

ANTAGONISTS OF CALCIUM

Even a diet adequate in calcium may fail to help under three circumstances: if the person gets too little vitamin D from the sun, food or supplements, eats too many foods with a high phosphorus content (taking in more phosphorus than calcium) or fails to secrete enough stomach acids to digest foods properly. Low secretion of hydrochloric acid is prevalent after people pass middle age.

A deficiency of hydrochloric acid (the medical name is hypochlorhydria) creates the same symptoms as a condition of excessive stomach acid.

"As we age, the parietal cells in the stomach lining produce less hydrochloric acid," writes Elizabeth Lipski, M.S., in *Digestive Wellness*. "In fact, half of the people over the age of 60 have hypochlorhydria . . . and by the age of 85, 80 percent of the healthy people tested had low stomach acid."[8]

Rather than just assuming that you have too little or too much stomach acid, ask your doctor to administer the Heidelberg Capsule Test, an accurate way of assessing what's going on in your stomach and removing the guesswork.

Individuals with a declining ability to secrete stomach acids can compensate by taking digestive enzymes that include hydrochloric acid. These are sold in all nutrition centers.

Authorities generally agree that the calcium intake should exceed that of phosphorus by two to two and a half to one. Individuals who eat a lot of eggs, meat, liver and other organ meats and consume many soft drinks—the latter have a high content of phosphoric acid—lose much of their ingested calcium. So do eaters of processed foods—"anything that comes in a bag, jar, can, wrapper or box," writes Sherry A. Rogers, M.D. "Phosphates are often not mentioned on the label or are listed under unrecognizable names as buffers, stabilizers, or acidifiers."[9]

"A high-phosphate diet also decreases the production of vitamin D (which already decreases with age) and is necessary for the incorporation of calcium into the bones," she concludes.

A calcium-rich diet can help most osteoporotic women—even when they are way up in years, as documented by an experiment at Kentucky State University.[10] Taken aback by the fact that 92 percent of women averaging 70 years of age had slight to marked osteoporosis, the researchers added three slices of cheese and three calcium tablets to the food of 20 of these patients for six months.

With an incredibly accurate measuring technique—quantitative radiography—they checked the density of the women's finger bones before *and* after the experiment. After six months, 11 of the 20 test subjects showed much greater bone density. Three retained the same level of bone—an impressive accomplishment in view of the usual rapid rate of bone loss in this critical period. The six remaining women lost some bone density; however, a total of 70 percent gained bone minerals or held their own.

THE REST OF THE TEAM

Although calcium is the most spectacular nutrient on the team—like the quarterback who gets most of the ink—this mineral needs all the rest of the players to do the job right. Vitamins and minerals you might never suspect have a major role in bone rebuilding:

vitamins A, B6, C, D and K, folic acid, and the minerals magnesium and manganese, boron, copper, silicon and zinc.[11]

Vitamin A helps to control the process of tearing down old bone cells and forming new ones. When your diet is short-changed on vitamin A, new bone cells are often formed faster than old cells can be evacuated. This causes abnormal bone formations which can bring on pain and—in the mouth—periodontal problems.

Likewise, vitamin B6 provides a strong support for good bone development. Several surveys give a less-than-subtle clue to why many women suffer from osteoporosis: almost one-half of supposedly healthy women are deficient in vitamin B6.

When generously supplied, vitamin B6 adds strength to connective tissue, the supporting structure of bones. It also seems to break down and neutralize homocysteine, a harmful substance which contributes not only to osteoporosis but also to cardiovascular complications.

There's even more. Vitamin B6 is a must for hydrochloric acid production, an absolute necessity for the absorption of calcium and for supporting function of the adrenal gland in secreting approximately 30 hormones, some of which help to maintain the blood's proper balance of minerals.

FOLIC ACID: A BIOCHEMICAL HERO

Another of the B vitamins, folic acid, also helps to transform the harmful homocysteine, which is derived from methionine, one of the eight essential amino acids.

Individuals with a genetic disorder in which large amounts of homocysteine accumulate are stricken with severe osteoporosis at an early age, as demonstrated by one study.[12] Before menopause, the body chemicals of women are efficient at converting homocysteine into less harmful substances. After that, they are not. This may account for rapid bone degeneration in postmenopausal women, say some authorities.

When methionine was given to premenopausal and postmenopausal women, the latter group showed a greater rise in homocysteine, which can also contribute to cardiovascular complications. A supplement of folic acid reduced the level of this harmful substance, although none of the volunteers tested showed a deficiency of folic acid.[13]

Researchers concluded that there seems to be a greater-than-average need for folic acid after menopause. If this need is not met, threatening homocysteine levels seem to rise. Studies disclose that 22 percent of individuals 65 years of age are folic-acid deficient.[14] Further, alcohol drinking, smoking and the taking of oral contraceptives all contribute to a deficiency of folic acid.[15]

VITAMIN C: A QUIET CONTRIBUTOR

What does vitamin C have to do with strong bones? More than you may believe. It holds our cells together—those in soft tissue and in bones. To make the cells stick together, the body produces a gluelike substance called collagen, the most plentiful body protein. Without a liberal supply of vitamin C, collagen can't be produced.

Collagen helps to keep us from coming unglued. Vitamin C-deprived guinea pigs showed only a two to three percent tissue content of collagen after 14 days. Guinea pigs which continued their usual intake of vitamin C had 14 to 16 percent collagen in their tissue.[16] Vitamin C also serves as a biochemical escort, making certain that calcium is delivered where needed.[17]

CALCIUM WON'T WORK WITHOUT VITAMIN D

In Texas, the term "Big D" stands for Dallas. In biochemistry, Big D stands for the vitamin that enables calcium to work its wonders. It increases the ability of our intestinal mucous membrane cells to absorb calcium.[18] It increases the depositing of calcium in our bones. It helps to withdraw minerals from our bones when our blood levels become too low in calcium and phosphorus.[19]

How important is vitamin D to strong bones? Back in times when people knew little about vitamin D, they failed to get enough of it from foods or from sunlight. Bones weren't strong enough to grow straight. Rickets developed. Result: bowlegs and knock-knees.

One of the most dramatic demonstrations of how important vitamin D is—from the sun, in this instance—resulted from a study among the elderly at the Chelsea Soldier's Home, not far from Boston.[20]

Even with calcium abundantly supplied, volunteers showed an acute calcium deficiency. Men involved in the study were required to remain indoors for seven weeks. And, amazingly, their ability to absorb calcium plummeted by 60 percent!

Best food sources of vitamin D are cod liver oil and oily parts of herring, salmon and sardines, butter, egg yolk and liver. It was once believed that the 400 International Units of vitamin D fortification claimed for each quart of milk was enough for our health needs.

Then Michael Holick, M.D., of Boston University School of Medicine, studied 13 brands of milk and found that less than one-third of the samples came within 20 percent of their stated amount of vitamin D: 400 I.U.[21]

The reason apparently is that Vitamin D is fat-soluble and sometimes is added too early, and then of course is skimmed off with the cream. Dr. Holick says that the undependability of vitamin D fortification is a strong argument for reforming milk inspection.

Sadly, too low a blood level of vitamin D is most common in the elderly—particularly women—due to less and less dietary intake, a decreased ability to absorb this nutrient, and too little exposure to sunlight or skyshine.

Once vitamin D is asorbed, it must be converted to its most active form, a process helped along by the minerals magnesium and boron.

THE K RATION

One of the best kept secrets in biochemistry is the fact that vitamin K, well-known for its contribution to blood clotting, is a star performer in promoting strong, solid, healthy bones.

Without it, bones couldn't be formed, repaired or rebuilt. Vitamin K makes possible the synthesizing of osteocalcin, a protein matrix on which calcium attaches itself to build new bone cells.[21] Osteocalcin is like the chicken wire nailed to the sides of a house so that plaster or stucco can grip the surface. Beyond this function, osteocalcin acts like a magnet to attract ions of calcium.[22]

Because vitamin K is plentiful in vegetables and because friendly intestinal bacteria synthesize it, many nutrition authorities assume that everybody's blood levels of vitamin K are adequate.

They may not be. This is revealed by new and super-accurate blood testing. Further, many people avoid eating vitamin K-rich vegetables or they take antibiotics which wipe out the friendly intestinal bacteria which synthesize it, along with the microbial enemies.

A research study conducted in the Netherlands indicated that postmenopausal women are not getting enough vitamin K in their diets.[23] Almost one-fourth of them excreted calcium at an alarming rate. When they took vitamin K supplementation, this loss was reduced by 33 percent. The researchers concluded from this that bone loss had either been stopped or slowed appreciably. Both negative and positive animal and human studies show the towering importance of vitamin K to our bones. Rats put on a vitamin K-deficient diet lost increased amounts of calcium in their urine.[24]

Healing of rabbits with bone fractures was speeded up when a vitamin K supplement was given, even though these animals were already on a diet with a high level of this vitamin.[25]

From a great variety of experiments, it is evident that a vitamin K supplement may indeed be a valuable supplement when dealing with osteoporosis and broken bones.

MINERAL MINUTE MEN

When bones are threatened by osteoporosis, the first thing most people think about is calcium—and so they should.

However, along with the calcium, other essential minerals must also be supplied: magnesium, manganese, boron, copper and zinc.

Magnesium, a neglected nutrient in the diet of Americans—particularly women—contributes to the making of solid, enduring bones by changing vitamin D to its active form and by activating an enzyme that helps to create new calcium crystals in the bones.

Concentration of magnesium in body cells and in bones was subnormal in 16 out of 19 women with osteoporosis. Calcium crystal formation in the 16 was defective.[26] This appears to make patients more likely to sustain fractures. Calcium crystals formed in the three women with adequate levels of magnesium were found to be normal.

Could magnesium deficiency be an important reason for widespread osteoporosis? Definitely. A recent Gallup survey reveals the frightening fact that 72 per cent of adult Americans fall short of the RDA for this mineral.[27] And, remember that the RDA is regarded by many biochemists as just a survival amount. Are you among that 72 percent?

Another alarming fact disclosed by the survey is that magnesium intake decreases as we age—at the point in life when we need it most!

"A potential magnesium deficiency is a matter of concern for many individuals of all ages, but for the elderly, it could be particularly serious," states Richard Rivlin, M.D., program director of the Clinical Nutrition Research Unit at Memorial Sloan-Kettering Cancer Center in New York. He continues:

> The prevalence of heart disease, diabetes and even leg cramps increases dramatically among older persons, and these are all health conditions in which magnesium deficiency has been found.
>
> The Gallup survey showed a high general awareness of the importance of nutrients such as vitamin C and calcium. But it is clear that consumers are largely unaware of the role of magnesium—a nutrient that is essential for the function of other minerals like calcium, as well as the normal operation of the heart and muscles.

MANGANESE: AN ESSENTIAL MINERAL

So far as solid bones are concerned, another unsung hero is manganese, a definite requirement for synthesizing connective tissue and structural material in both cartilage and bone, and for assuring that needed minerals will remain in the bones.

When rats were fed a manganese-deficient diet, their bones were smaller, less mineral-dense and more subject to fracture than those of animals fed enough of this trace mineral.[28]

It was discovered that osteoporotic women had had only one-quarter of the manganese blood levels of women who were osteoporosis-free.[29]

BRING ON THE BORON!

Until recent years, even leading biochemists had no idea that the trace mineral boron could be useful anywhere in human nutrition, let alone in the bones.

One particular experiment rocked them like an earthquake. When an intake of three milligrams of boron was added to the typical daily diet of post-menopausal women, the amount of calcium which they excreted in urine dropped by a dramatic 44 percent.[30]

At the same time, their blood serum concentration of the most biologically active form of estrogen rose sharply—to the same level as in the women receiving estrogen therapy.

How does boron accomplish such a remarkable thing? Biochemists can only offer an educated guess. When boron joins certain organic chemicals, it appears to promote the synthesis of the most usable form of estrogen.

It is well established that estrogen therapy for osteoporosis in postmenopausal women—synthetic hormones are used—poses danger of certain cancers: cervical and breast. Does this mean that boron presents the same risk? Not at all, say authorities.

Oral estrogen must be taken in relatively high doses to clear the intestinal tract and reach the bloodstream in effective form. In contrast, the amount of estrogen produced with the help of boron is only about five percent of the oral dose. Therefore, it produces the desired effect with virtually no cancer risk.[31]

Just as boron helps in synthesizing a form of estrogen which contributes to bone integrity, it appears also to help in turning vitamin D into its most useful form. In an experiment with chicks, boron deficiency worsened a vitamin D deficiency and made for abnormally formed bones.[32]

A daily intake of only three milligrams of boron appears to bring about dramatic changes in bone formation and strength, according to U.S. Department of Agriculture studies.

THE COPPER QUESTION

As with boron, just a trace of copper is necssary to promote and maintain solid bone structure. A mere three mg daily is generally recommended. (More is not better so far as trace minerals are concerned. In fact, more can be dangerous.) Surveys indicate that the diet of most people includes only about one mg of copper daily—about a third of the required amount.

Even authorities in nutrition don't know exactly

how copper works on body bones, but they are aware of several rat studies which demonstrate that a copper deficiency permits the escape of significant amounts of bone minerals and, therefore, contributes to the weakening of bones.

SILICON: SUPER MINERAL

Another essential mineral which many doctors forget to include in the osteoporotic's diet is silicon. Only in the last few decades has it become known that silicon is an essential nutrient, particularly for sound bones and teeth.

A great deal of research demonstrates that silicon is of paramount importance in forming cartilage and other connective tissue. Silicon is found in heavy concentrations in early stages of bone calcification.

Animals deficient in silicon show abnormalities of bone formation, especially in the skull.

Frank Murray, in the *Big Family Guide to All the Minerals,* writes:

"In laboratory studies, Edith M. Carlisle, Ph.D, of the School of Public Health, University of California at Los Angeles, has determined that silicon plays an important role in connective tissue and, notably, in bone and cartilage. Both abnormalities of bone and cartilage have shown up in silicon-deficient animals."[33]

GET IN SYNC WITH ZINC!

Noted for its contributions to wound healing, to a smooth and healthy skin and to normal gland function—including that of the thymus, the immune system's key gland—zinc gets little recognition for its part in assuring bone health.

However, zinc is needed to enhance vitamin D's efficiency in fostering calcium absorption, for bone to form normally and for putting the brakes on a too-rapid loss of bone minerals, especially in the jawbone.[34]

Deficiency of zinc could be one of the major causes of osteoporosis, inasmuch as several surveys show that people take in too little zinc. Further, many authorities judge that the RDA for this mineral is too low.

Several reports disclose that "substantial portions of the U.S. population may be at risk of a zinc deficiency." Certain population groups are at especially high risk: infants, young children, the elderly, the pregnant, the nursing and alcoholics.

Michael Lesser, M.D., in addressing the Senate Select Committee on Nutrition and Human Needs, stated that the soil of 32 states is zinc-deficient and that universally used commercial fertilizers return no zinc to the earth.[35]

Several U.S. Department of Agriculture surveys show the same thing. It is impossible for even a magician to pull a rabbit out of a hat without first having put one inside. Another study revealed that the blood and bones of elderly osteoporosis patients were deficient in zinc.[36]

Added to that, all forms of zinc are not created equal. Some are hard to absorb. Zinc picolinate seems to be the form of zinc most readily absorbed, transported, assimilated and used by the body.

AMOUNTS OF NEEDED SUPPLEMENTS

We've already considered the body's requirements for the mineral calcium. However, let's review the RDA (Required Daily Allowance) for vitamins A, B6, C, D and K and folic acid, as well as the minerals magnesium, manganese, boron, copper, silicon and zinc—all needed to build better bones—and decide if they are adequate. Then let's read the list of foods which contain the greatest amounts of these nutrients.

The RDA for vitamin A is 5000 International Units for men and women. (Most authorities feel that 10,000 I.U. is an unsafe amount for pregnant women, inasmuch as their babies may suffer various malformations.)

Foods richest in *vitamin A* are calves' liver, egg yolk, swordfish, whitefish and various cheeses. Some nutritionists count the amounts of beta-carotene in foods as vitamin A. However, this is not always the case. Although beta-carotene is a vitamin A precursor, it needs to be translated into vitamin A by the liver. When the liver's function is inefficient—as in a deficiency of thyroid hormone—it can't convert beta carotene into vitamin A.

Here are the foods with the greatest amounts of provitamin A (beta carotene): dandelion greens, collard greens, carrots, yams, red peppers, winter squash and, among others, cantaloupe, apricots and broccoli.

The RDA for *vitamin B6* is 2 to 2.5 mg for adults. It is difficult to find this vitamin in such low potencies. Generally, vitamin B6 is present in B-complex capsules or tablets in potencies of 25, 50, and 100 mg. Excesses are thrown off.

Best food and supplement sources of vitamin B-6 are brewer's yeast, brown rice, whole wheat, royal jelly, soybeans, rye, lentils, sunflower seeds and hazelnuts.

Folic acid's RDA for adults is 400 to 800 micrograms. The richest supplement and food sources are torula yeast, brewer's yeast, alfalfa, soybeans, endive, chickpeas, oats, lentils and wheat germ. Vegetables and fruits also contain liberal amounts.

The RDA for *vitamin C* is 50 to 80 mg for adults. Many biochemists feel that the proper daily amount could range anywhere from 100 mg to 10,000 mg. At high potencies, this vitamin sometimes has a laxative effect at first.

Supplements and foods rating highest in vitamin C content are rose hips, acerola cherries, guavas, black currants, green peppers, chives, kiwi fruit, strawberries and citrus fruits.

The RDA for *vitamin D* is 400 I.U. A quart of

vitamin D-fortified milk is said to contain this amount, but a study mentioned earlier questions this claim.

Supplements and foods richest in vitamin D are cod and other fish liver oils, sardines, salmon, tuna, mushrooms, shrimp, sunflower seeds, liver, eggs and butter.

No RDA has been established for *vitamin K*. However, biochemists generally agree that 300 micrograms is an adequate intake. More than 500 mcg of the synthetic form of vitamin K is considered toxic.

Although vitamin K is noted for coming mainly from vegetables and fruit, the foods with the richest K content are two cheeses: cheddar and camembert. Brussels sprouts, soy lecithin, alfalfa, oats, spinach, soybeans, cauliflower, cabbage and broccoli all have a high content of this nutrient.

Now for the minerals:

The RDA for *calcium* is 800 mg for adults. Many nutritionists believe that this is low and that 1000 to 1600 mg would be a more realistic range.

Dairy products would seem to be at the top of the list for the richest calcium content, but this is not so. It is, therefore, easy for those who avoid milk, butter, cheese and yogurt to find excellent alternates, some even richer in calcium by volume. Sesame seeds and kelp are the leaders. Then come various cheeses, brewer's yeast, sardines, carob, caviar (for those with a thick wallet or heavy purse), soybeans, almonds and brazil nuts.

Magnesium's RDA is 350 mg for men and 450 mg for women. Usually magnesium intake is at a 1:2 ratio with that of calcium. So 1000 mg of calcium would call for 500 mg of magnesium. Some authorities now insist that magnesium intake should be equal to that of calcium.

Supplements and foods richest in magnesium are kelp, blackstrap molasses, sunflower seeds, wheat germ, almonds, soybeans, brazil nuts, soy lecithin and hazelnuts.

The RDA for *manganese* is five mgs. Surprisingly, tea leaves contain the richest supply of this trace mineral. Ginger, buckwheat, oats, hazelnuts, chestnuts, wheat, pecans, barley, sunflower seeds, ginseng and watercress follow.

A safe *boron* intake has been established by the U.S. Department of Agriculture as three mgs, an amount accepted by most biochemists. Foods with the highest boron content are soybeans, almonds, peanuts, raisins, dates, unprocessed honey and all the fruits and vegetables.

Although *copper* has no established RDA, various experts suggest that two to three mgs daily is an acceptable range. An excess of the higher amount could upset the zinc-to-copper ratio.

Mushrooms, liver, oysters, mussels, wheat germ, blackstrap molasses, lobster, honey, hazelnuts, brazil nuts, walnuts, kelp, salmon and cashews are best bets for copper content.

The RDA for *zinc* is 15 to 25 mg for adults. Oysters are a virtual treasury of zinc, but they are best avoided because they live in polluted environments and are among the greatest garbage collectors of the sea. After oysters in the ratings come herring, sesame seeds, torula yeast, blackstrap molasses, maple syrup, liver, soybeans, sunflower seeds, egg yolk, lamb, chicken, cocoa and brewer's yeast.

Silicon has no established RDA. Organ meats, whole grains, algae and the herb horsetail are the best sources of silicon.

ೞ 5 ೞ

GET MORE MILEAGE
OUT OF YOUR CALCIUM

A new patient, a postmenopausal woman with the beginnings of osteoporosis, complained to me that the calcium tablets her previous physician had recommended were doing her no good.

Once I learned her brand, I said, "You may be right. I happened to test that brand of calcium myself and found that it dissolves so slowly that it goes through you without offering any help.

"That's what I call tourist calcium. It makes a pleasant trip down the alimentary canal and is gone."

THE SHANGRAW STUDY

I told her results of the one-year calcium product study of Ralph Shangraw, University of Maryland professor of pharmaceutics. One out of every three calcium pills leaves the stomach before it can take effect. Eleven of 35 calcium carbonate supplements tested took so long to disintegrate that they were eliminated before they could do any good.[1]

Only 17 products dissolved within the time period when they could be useful. The standard set by the United States Pharmacopeia (USP) is 30 minutes. Just 14 disintegrated in 10 minutes or less—excellent time.

"Nutritional supplements aren't required by law to meet USP standards," says Shangraw. He advises us to use nationally advertised brands, many of which dissolve within ten minutes. The authors use capsules of finely ground particles of calcium.

So that you can be satisfied that you have an effective product, Shangraw advises checking with your pharmacist for his or her recommendation or testing your calcium yourself. Drop a calcium tablet into a glass of vinegar. It has to disintegrate in 30 minutes or less—the faster, the better. If it doesn't, you need another brand.

A SUCCESSFUL ALTERNATIVE

An alternate procedure is to take a supplement of microcrystalline hydroxyapatite (MCHC), capsules of fine crystals of raw bone concentrate. It is well assimilable and contains every ingredient needed for bone building.

At the University of Florida, 250 women with osteoporosis took part in a study. One third of the women received a placebo that looked like a supplement for bone building. To another third was administered calcium gluconate. And the remaining third were given microcrystalline hydroxyapatite.[2]

The group which received the placebo showed significant bone demineralization. Those who took calcium gluconate held their own—no gain, no loss. However, the group taking microcrystalline hydroxyapatite had an impressive gain in bone thickness: 6.1 percent.

DOWN WITH MILK!

Today the dietary accent seems to be on increasing use of low-fat or no-fat dairy products as an effective calcium source. The anti-dairy products group utters a resounding and passionate NO! It calls for using vegetarian sources of calcium, which are supposedly more readily absorbable.

Of course, many people are milk intolerant, partially or totally unable to process lactose (milk sugar) because they lack the digestive enzyme lactase. Others may be allergic to milk and suffer the symptoms generally accompanying allergies: watering eyes, sneezing, wheezing, an outbreak of rash or generalized itching.

Dr. Sherry Rogers makes the point that eating a great deal of cheese often adds unwanted calories and consequent weight gain. The phosphorus content of dairy products is also too high relative to calcium. She states that one ounce of cheese contains 204 milligrams of calcium and 115 calories. However, a stalk of broccoli contains 215 mg of calcium and just 50 calories. Broccoli provides much more magnesium, manganese and boron, she observes.[3]

Nutrition-oriented physician Alan R. Gaby agrees with Dr. Rogers about the advantage of some greens over milk in terms of calcium quantity and bioavailability.[4]

VEGETARIAN CALCIUM BETTER ABSORBED

In the *Townsend Letter for Doctors,* Dr. Gaby writes that absorption of 300 mg of calcium from kale was measured in 11 women and compared with their absorption of calcium from milk. Their mean absorption from kale was 40.9 percent, compared with 32.1 percent from milk.

Dr. Gaby's commentary follows:

Many dark green leafy vegetables are known to have a relatively high calcium concentration. The calcium in spinach, however, is poorly absorbed, presumably because of its high concentration of oxalate. The present study demonstrates that kale, a low-oxalate vegetable, is a good source of bioavailable calcium.

Kale is one of the varieties of *Brassica oleracea,* which includes broccoli, turnip greens, collard greens, and mustard greens. These low oxalate, calcium-rich vegetables are, therefore, also likely to be good sources of bioavailable calcium. Milk is believed to be a contributing factor in the etiology of atherosclerosis and many allergic and autoimmune disorders. A safer source of dietary calcium is therefore desirable for some individuals.

In some of her lectures, the late Adelle Davis dramatized the importance of calcium by saying that "without it, our bones would be so soft that they could be tied in knots like ropes of modeling clay."

As it is, our bones are as strong as steel—and far lighter—and resilient enough to take a sudden sharp impact, assuming they have a rich content of calcium and the trace minerals and vitamins mentioned earlier.

TIMING FOR CALCIUM IS IMPORTANT

One aspect of calcium taking is little considered by most people: the time of day when it is best absorbed. Morris Notelovitz, professor of obstetrics and gynecology at the University of Florida, has done a great deal of research on this subject and consequently is one of the nation's leading authorities in this area.[5]

Calcium is best absorbed when it is needed the most. "During the day we get calcium from our food and fluids such as milk and from other dairy products. At night, there's no such intake, because we're sleeping and not eating or drinking. However, the body still needs a certain amount of calcium in the blood.

"What happens then? The body takes calcium from the only available source—the bones, where calcium is the major mineral."

BEDTIME THE BEST TIME FOR CALCIUM

There are two main reasons why it is best to take calcium right at bedtime.

"First, existing calcium levels are low, so absorption of this supplement is both rapid and successful. Second, at night time, you are not taking in other food which can interfere with calcium's absorption.

"Such timing for calcium supplementation can help to prevent osteoporosis, the bone-thinning and weakening degenerative disease that affects some 16 million older Americans—particularly women."

Dr. Notelovitz adds that it's not a good idea to take a calcium supplement on an empty stomach. "It's best to have a glass of milk or another calcium-containing food first."

One of Dr. Notelovitz's ways of enriching the diet with calcium is by adding powdered, nonfat dry milk to beverages, casseroles and soups. Each teaspoon adds 50 milligrams, he claims. Relative to soups, he recommends adding a dash of vinegar when you are preparing stock from bones to dissolve their calcium. One pint of soup made in this manner will have as much calcium as a quart of milk, he states.

Of course, natural sources of calcium offer the most benefits. However, when buying a calcium supplement, how can you tell which types offer the greatest advantages? Here's the response of Abram Hoffer, M.D., one of the best known alternative physicians:

"Heaney examined the bioavailability of different calcium sources. He and his colleagues found that absorption from all sources, natural and supplements, is about the same."

Then he makes the following point:

"However, there is a difference in absorption when calcium sources are taken with water only or with food. With food, even with lack of HCL (hydrochloric acid), absorption is about the same. As with all supplements, calcium sources are best taken with food."[6]

AVOID SOFT WATER FOR DRINKING!

One of the little-known sources of extra calcium and magnesium in the diet is hard drinking water. Hardness in water comes from calcium and magnesium.

Through the years, numerous studies have shown that bone diseases such as osteoporosis rarely occur in areas where the water is hard. It is the same for heart attacks and strokes.

In a Wisconsin study of 1,400 farmers, those who drank hard water from their wells had a neglible amount of heart attacks and strokes compared with farmers who drank soft water.[7] Individuals who have water-softening devices in their homes for better washing of clothing and dishes and better bathing often drink the soft water and, therefore, make themselves more vulnerable to heart attacks and strokes as well as to osteoporosis.

Health-aware people use a two-source system to give them access to soft water for washing and hard water for drinking.

❧ 6 ❧

THE ESTROGEN DILEMMA

In the mid-1960s Dr. Robert Wilson created a seismic sensation with his best-selling book *Feminine Forever,* which told menopausal women that, with estrogen replacement therapy (ERT), they could banish hot flashes, weepiness, headaches, nervousness and inability to sleep and—best of all!—stay young.

Hazards of ERT were soft-pedaled. Consequently, millions of women followed the Wilson regimen, some of them with eventual regrets when they experienced adverse reactions such as breast or cervical cancer.

Approximately 10 years later Sheldon H. Cherry, M.D., an obstetrician and gynecologist at Mount Sinai Hospital in New York City, attacked the Wilson thesis, stating that estrogen didn't keep women young and feminine forever. Female longevity, in many instances, was actually reduced, because taking estrogen sometimes caused them to develop serious medical ailments, including cancer.

THE TRUTH ABOUT MENOPAUSE

In a slender paperback, *The Menopause Myth,* Dr. Cherry stated that many symptoms associated with menopause should have been dissociated, because they had more to do with factors not directly related to menopause: children leaving the nest, husbands being more preoccupied with careers than with their wives, and the feeling of vanishing attractiveness and youthfulness.

"There are only two types of menopausal symptoms," Dr. Cherry told Ursula Vils, a *Los Angeles Times* reporter.[1] "One group is called the vasomotor symptoms, which are hot flashes and sweats. The other is vaginal atrophy—in lay terms, the drying and thinning of the skin that would result in pain during intercourse or itching and burning.

"A lot of other symptoms have been confused with menopause, such as depression, insomnia, nervousness, weepiness, rapid heartbeat and headaches," he continued. "These are all anxiety and depressive symptoms that women can get at any time of their lives. Women tend to get them at this time for a number of reasons that I think are culturally determined, that are peculiar to our American society."

Only 20 percent of the women have severe menopausal symptoms, Cherry maintained. Some women should be put on estrogen replacement therapy. However, they should be made aware of its risks.

"Menopause is not a deficiency disease," he stated. "And estrogen is not a panacea, it is not the elixer of youth. It is downright dangerous."

THE ESTROGEN FACTOR

After menopause, estrogen production sharply declines and bone loss consequently, increases. Borje E.C. Nordin, of the Royal Adelaide Hospital in Adelaide, Australia, discovered much lower estrogen levels in postmenopausal women with osteoporosis than in healthy postmenopausal women.[2]

Dr. Robert Lindsay, an osteoporosis authority at Helen Hayes Hospital in West Haverstraw, New York, conducted an experiment which revealed that estrogen replacement can prevent spinal fractures— medical nightmares—in healthy postmenopausal women.[3]

Yet many medical doctors who favor estrogen therapy for preventing or slowing osteoporosis do not routinely prescribe it for this purpose, because it poses a risk of uterine and, possibly, even breast cancer. Conscientious and responsible doctors make patients aware of the risk factors. Adding progestin to the orthodox hormone treatment has lessened the cancer risk slightly, but hasn't eliminated it.

THE ESTROGEN BATTLEGROUND

Like a shuttlecock in a badminton game, the issue has been swatted back and forth. Some authorities claim that estrogen lessens the chances of abnormal blood clotting and heart attacks. Others claim it promotes heart disease.

Some authorities quote statistics which say that ERT contributes to breast and endometrial cancer. Others quote statistics that show the opposite. Just more than a decade ago, two studies appeared back to back in the *New England Journal of Medicine*. One stated that estrogen prevents heart disease. The other insisted that it causes heart disease.[4]

Inasmuch as both studies were found valid by the editors and referees, the journal published both. Researchers at the Framingham Heart Study, a long-running survey of the health of members of one community—1,234 postmenopausal women were studied—revealed that the risk of heart attack was twice as high among estrogen-taking women, as among nontakers.

A Harvard Medical School survey of 121,964 postmenopausal female nurses compared the number of heart attacks and fatal heart disease of estrogen takers and nontakers. Conclusion? The risk of heart disease was one-third as high among estrogen users.

Synthetic estrogen for postmenopausal women differs from the natural hormone, which cannot be taken orally, because digestive juices break it down.

In *Preventing and Reversing Osteoporosis,* Alan R. Gaby, M.D. reminds us that there are three kinds of estrogen which can help with osteoporosis. The first two—estrone and estradiol—are potent and could be hazardous to health, and the third, estriol, which occurs naturally in the body, does not cause cancer and has even shown some anticancer activity.[5]

THE CANCER QUESTION

A study of more than 118,000 female nurses over a 10-year period disclosed that women who take estrogen are 35 to 40 percent more likely to develop cancer, stated researcher Graham Colditz, of Boston's Brigham and Women's Hospital, in a 1990 Associated Press story. Colditz suggested that women weigh the risks versus the benefits of estrogen replacement therapy and pointed out that "a very large study published in *The New England Journal of Medicine,* assessing risk factors for hip fractures in white women, which followed over 9500 women for eight years, found no benefit in estrogen supplementation in women over the age of 65."[6]

Colditz added that once women stop taking estrogen, the risk is eliminated, good news for women who have used this form of hormone therapy. Further, progestin, a synthetic hormone, is now widely taken with estrogen for protection against cancer and other side effects.

CONSEQUENCES OF OVARIAN SURGERY

Harry K. Genant, M.D., professor of radiology, medicine and orthopedics at the University of California at San Francisco, made a thorough survey of the critical problem of rapid bone loss after menopause.

Bone loss in the spine of women whose ovaries had been surgically removed was frighteningly rapid: 7 to 9 percent annually on average.[7] Some women lost as much as 15 to 20 percent.

Genant's research with the spine was the first of its kind and also revealed that women who go through menopause naturally lose bone minerals more slowly than women with surgically-induced menopause: 5 percent annually, still a threatening rate.[8]

The cancer threat is real, because Genant's study disclosed that only a high dose of estrogen—0.6 mg—could manage osteoporosis. Five out of six patients lost no bone on the 0.6 mg dosage and some even recovered a small amount of bone minerals.

DOES ERT WORK?

Does estrogen replacement therapy actually promote new bone formation? Alan Gaby, M.D., who has analyzed numerous studies, tells us that estrogen slows the rate of bone loss, but does not increase bone formation. In some cases, it actually causes a slight bone loss.[9]

In her no-punches-pulled *Menopause: A Positive Approach*, Rosetta Reitz reveals the bald facts about estrogen replacement therapy:

"In spite of the threatening promise by the estrogen-pushers that estrogen replacement therapy (ERT) can 'prevent,' 'relieve,' 'cure,' and 'correct' osteoporosis, it has been clearly stated by Dr. Heaney [a world authority on osteoporosis] at the biggest conference on menopause and aging . . . that 'plainly estrogens have not proved successful in treatment of osteoporosis.'"[10]

Best-selling writer Earl Mindell, R.Ph., Ph.D., in *What You Should Know About Natural Health For Women,* writes:

"There is no question that estrogen can slow bone loss around the time of menopause, but the scientific evidence is very clear that after five or six years, bone loss continues at the same rate, with or without estrogen."[11]

An osteoporosis authority, Dr. Robert Lindsay, professor of clinical medicine at Columbia University College of Physicians and Surgeons, casts his vote in favor of estrogen for osteoporosis, stating that at least 10 studies show that estrogen therapy reduces the risk of all fractures.[12]

"Specifically estrogen therapy reduces the danger of vertebral, wrist and hip fractures by at least 50 percent. Even when given to women with established osteoporosis, estrogens prevent further bone loss and reduce by half the risk of recurrent vertebral fractures.

"Recent evidence suggests that the earlier treatment is begun and the longer it is continued, the greater the benefit. The maximum effects of estrogens are obtained while patients are still taking them."

To reduce the risk of possible cancer of the endometrium or breasts, he suggests that doctors use progestin sequentially with estrogen for at least 12 days or also give it in combination with estrogen.

THREAT FROM ENVIRONMENTAL POLLUTION

Several authorities ponder the wisdom of estrogen replacement therapy in view of increasing environmental pollution with fat-soluble, non-biologically degradable pesticides which mimic estrogen and would add to the hormone burden and possibly increase the chance of negative side effects.

The consequences? Diminished sperm production, infertility and testicular cancer in males, shown in human beings and animals, and increased hormone-related breast disease, uterine and vaginal cancers in women. Pesticides banned in the United States are sometimes exported to foreign nations—often Third World countries—and returned to us in imported food products or on upper atmosphere winds. Several studies show that pesticides used in Central America are carried many thousands of miles away—as far as Lake Michigan in the Middle West.

Environmental chemicals "can mimic hormones and rearrange genes," writes Sherry A. Rogers, M.D.

PROGESTERONE INSTEAD OF ESTROGEN

Dr. Alan Gaby wonders why today's doctors concentrate so heavily on administering estrogen to postmenopausal women to combat osteoporosis, rather than the hormone progesterone, also produced by the ovaries.

Progesterone is much safer than estrogen and may be more effective in coping with osteoporosis, he writes. (Progesterone is the natural hormone; progestin is the synthetic version.)

A comprehensive study by Jerilynn C. Price, M.D., of the division of Endocrinology and Metabolism at the University of British Columbia, shows that progesterone definitely builds new and stronger bones.[13]

This is borne out by an in-depth study of 100

postmenopausal women—from ages 38 to 83, averaging 65.2—by John R. Lee, M.D., of Sebastopol, California. These women applied to their skin a cream containing 3 percent progesterone.[14]

A majority had already shown a marked shortening of stature, indication of one or more spontaneous vertebral fractures. When appropriate, Dr. Lee administered conjugated estrogens—such as Premarin—0.3 to 0.625 milligrams daily.

However, approximately 35 percent of the women were unable to take estrogen, because of medical conditions which would have made estrogen replacement too hazardous to their health: breast disease, a history of breast cancer, blood clotting disorders, thromboembolism, fibrocystic breast disease, endometrial cancer, high cholesterol or triglyceride levels, or varicose veins.

For a minimum of three years, all volunteers applied the progesterone cream for 12 consecutive nights monthly or during the last two weeks of estrogen use. To assure efficient absorption, the cream was applied on a rotation basis, to soft skin areas—under the arms, or on the face or neck.

Dr. Lee recommended that volunteers also increase their intake of leafy green vegetables, take nutritional supplements daily—including vitamins C and D and calcium—minimize the use of alcohol, cigarettes or red meat, and perform aerobic exercise three times weekly.

The results highlighted the importance of progesterone in the war with osteoporosis. Decline in height stopped and stabilized, pains in bones and muscles disappeared, and no additional fractures occurred.

However, the most exciting progress was manifested in comparative bone density. Sixty-three of the 100 were able to afford bone density studies—by means of dual photon absorptiometry—every three to six months. Inasmuch as the remaining 37 women had neither the personal money nor insurance coverage to pay for the tests, they declined them.

Over three years, the predicted average bone loss should have been 4.5 percent. Yet, among the 63 treated with progesterone, in whom bone density was continually measured, every one showed an increase in bone mass by an average of 15.4 percent. Such a dramatic increase in bone mass has not been achieved by means of any other osteoporosis treatment! Seventy-year-old women showed the same gains as younger ones, leading to the conclusion that it's never too late to start this therapy, despite the degree of bone deterioration.

ANOTHER ALTERNATIVE

Although estrogen treatment, combined with progestin, is perhaps the most commonly used therapy of orthodox doctors, a close second is administration of calcitonin, which is a natural secretion of the parathyroid glands, whose job it is to regulate the metabolism of calcium and phosphorus. The parathyroid glands—four units in a cluster—are located right next to the thyroid gland or embedded in it. Some of the parathyroid glands' actions are similar to those of estrogen.

In the manner of estrogen, salmon calcitonin (the most commonly administered calcitonin) blocks the action of osteoclasts, cells that cause bone breakdown and absorption. In human anatomy, women are short-changed by nature in the amount of calcitonin which they can secrete. Not so men.

Usually administered subcutaneously (under the skin), salmon calcitonin now is available as a nasal spray which delivers a 200 I.U. dosage and is usually given daily, states Dr. Robert Lindsay. The spray dosage is somewhat weaker than the subcutaneous form, and the spray treatment costs approximately $2.00 per day.[15]

Several studies show that postmenopausal women with osteoporosis have a lower amount of calcitonin reserve than nonosteoporotic women and that taking calcitonin has increased the bone mass of women *and* men.

Calcitonin, injected under the skin or into a muscle, is probably the most expensive treatment for osteoporosis. Rapid price changes make it impossible to give an accurate cost estimate.

Although effective, calcitonin causes quickly-passing face flushing—as does the B vitamin niacin—

nausea, sometimes with vomiting, in a small percentage of patients. On rare occasions, it causes severe allergic reactions—even anaphylactic shock—and, in one instance, brought on death. Still doctors generally consider calcitonin a fairly safe drug.

CONSIDER ETIDRONATE

Another synthetic drug that blocks bone destruction and absorption is etidronate, which is a chemical look-alike of pyrophosphate, a combination of phosphorus and carbon made naturally by the body.

In a two-year study, 429 postmenopausal women with osteoporosis and fractures of the vertebrae were given either etidronate or a placebo.[16] Those receiving etidronate showed base bone increases across the board—4.4 to 5.2 percent gains in bone mass of the lumbar spine and smaller increases in bone mass at the hip. Also, those supplemented with etidronate experienced a significant reduction in subsequent fractures compared with the others. Volunteers on the placebo showed a serious bone loss and a high incidence of fractures after the study.

Presently etidronate is not approved by the Food and Drug Administration (FDA) for osteoporosis, although authorized for treatment of a severe bone disorder called Paget's disease and for abnormal calcium deposits which sometimes follow hip replacement surgery.

Yet nothing stops a medical doctor from prescribing an FDA-approved drug for another purpose, if such a modality seems appropriate for the medical condition.

Cost of etidronate is somewhat lower than that of calcitonin, and this drug is virtually free of side effects.

Other effective agents in preventing bone loss are the bisphosphonates. They are usually poorly absorbed through the intestinal tract. Alendronate, the only FDA-approved bisphosphonate at this date, is best absorbed with eight ounces of water upon arising before any food, beverage or medication is consumed. The patient should not lie down or eat or drink anything for at least 30 minutes after drinking it. The daily dosage suggested by Dr. Lindsay is 10 mg, which, at this writing, costs approximately $1.50 to $2.00.[17]

Dr. Lindsay cites results from using alendronate in Phase III clinical studies—extreme cases:

Alendronate produced an approximate 8 percent increase in vertebral bone mass over three years and a smaller increase in femoral neck bone mass. This was associated with a 50 percent reduction in vertebral fracture.

Data presented at the recent World Congress on Osteoporosis in Amsterdam indicated that alendronate reduces the risk of hip fracture by about 50 percent and the risk of vertebral fracture by about 80 percent.

Dr. Lindsay characterizes alendronate as an effective agent for the treatment of osteoporosis, but concludes with a warning: "The long-term consequences of the presence of bisphosphonates in the skeleton are unknown."

FLUORIDE TREATMENT INEFFECTIVE

Fluoride does not live up to its reputation in osteoporosis treatment. A dose of 30 mg a day has been demonstrated in some studies to increase bone mass of osteoporotics. However, the new bone is of low to moderate quality, prone to possible fractures.

Sometimes the side effects of fluoride treatment are not reported in the popular media. Yet they are real and numerous and serious enough to make us hesitant to try it, when more beneficial and less risky treatments are available.

Fluoride's most serious side effects are anemia, arthritis, gastrointestinal upsets and recurrent vomiting.

∾ 7 ∾

EXERCISE FOR BONE BUILDING

Several studies indicate that how you exercise is as important to preventing, neutralizing or reversing osteoporosis as how you eat.

All right. What are the exercise best bets?

Jogging, running or tennis, state Peter Jacobson and associates at the University of North Carolina in Chapel Hill, who have done much experimentation in this field.[1]

Doctors who advocate an exercise program for osteoporotics issue a red-flag warning. Some osteoporosis has gone so far that exercise might cause bone collapse, so it's best to have your doctor check you carefully before approving an exercise program.

Jacobson says that weight-bearing exercise can often counter bone loss after menopause.[2] He compared postmenopausal women who played tennis three times a week with age-matched nonexercising women. The tennis players had much more bone mass than the sedentary women, accenting the fact that exercise can slow or prevent bone loss.

BEST BONE-BULDING EXERCISES

Aerobic dancing not only melts off surplus suet, it is also a phenomenal activity for coping with osteoporosis, as discovered by R. Bruce Martin, director of orthopedic research at the West Virginia Medical Center.[3]

Martin and co-workers tested several exercises on middle-aged women, the prime test volunteers, because bone demineralizes most rapidly in the ten years following menopause.

One group did aerobic dancing. A second group walked two miles a day four times a week. A third group's only exercise was avoiding exercise. "Before" and "after" tests made a striking impression on researchers—on patients, too. After six months, the nonexercisers had lost 1.5 percent of their calcium and other major minerals in arm bone.

The walkers, too, lost some bone minerals, but not quite as much. However, the aerobic dancers lost none of the key minerals in the arm bone, supposedly because they exercised both arms and legs. The dancers and walkers showed a marked gain: greater width of the arm bone.

DOING THE IMPOSSIBLE: REVERSING OSTEOPOROSIS

An excellent way to to beat osteoporosis is by exercising regularly, states Everett L. Smith, Ph.D., an authority on the biology of aging at the University of Wisconsin in Madison. And he has the statistics to prove it.[4] Combining exercise with supernutrition builds better bones faster.

Dr. Smith discovered that the throwing arm of young baseball pitchers and the arm swinging a tennis racket have much more bone mineral mass than the other arm. He also studied older tennis players—those averaging 64 years of age—and found the identical condition in their dominant arm.

Then he concentrated on 38 women who were an average 84 years old, dividing them into two groups: 18 nonexercisers and 12 who performed physical activity half an hour each week for three years. Each exerciser sat on a chair and performed 103 different movements, motions calculated to utilize most of the body bones.

Three years later, the nonexercisers showed a loss of 3.29 percent of their bone minerals. In sharp contrast, the exercisers revealed a gain of 2.29 percent of the bone mineral content. The Smith experiment tends to show it's never too late to battle osteoporosis—and win!

WEIGHT-BEARING EXERCISE IS BEST

Repeated physical stress applied to the bones is supposed to be the way that weight-bearing exercise stops or reverses osteoporosis. Pressure is put on the bones by the force of muscular contraction or body weight in simple activities such as walking, jogging, running, bouncing on a trampoline, or playing tennis or basketball.

Swimming has not been regarded a good exercise for weight losing or preventing osteoporosis, although excellent for the cardiovascular system. However, recent studies weaken this notion.

Men from ages 40 to 83, whose only exercise was competitive swimming, showed a significantly larger bone mass in the forearm and vertebrae compared with nonexercisers.

Something similar happened to women swimmers ranging in age from 37 years old to seniors. They increased vertebral bone density by daily sessions in the pool—much more than nonswimmers.

Dr. Alan Gaby sums up the considerable value of swimming in staying ahead of osteoporosis.[5]

"While swimming does not increase bone density as much as weight-bearing exercises, it does have a beneficial effect on bone mass. This finding is important, because some elderly individuals with osteoporosis are too frail to perform weight-bearing exercises. For them, swimming can be a gentle, nontraumatic way to increase bone mass."

Couch potatoes who spend hours on the sofa watching TV are unwittingly contributing to their bone loss—particularly the middle-aged and elderly. There are big benefits to giving up the horizontal life for the vertical.

Numerous studies demonstrate that our bone mass and density are directly related to the amount of physical exercise we perform. One study of 48 postmenopausal women revealed that physically fit exercisers had greater bone mineral content in the thigh bone and the lumbar spine than women of the same age who were less physically fit.[6]

BUT I'M TOO OLD TO EXERCISE!

Many people who are not seriously ill actually talk themselves into developing osteoporosis with the excuse that "I'm too old to exercise." Just the idea of giving up exercise subconsciously tells these persons they are too old for physical activities and hurries the aging process.

Of course, it is essential for them to have a complete physical exam by their doctor to determine their fitness. Even bedridden individuals can stave off osteoporosis by arm exercises which any physician can prescribe.

One of my chronic patients renewed his energy and life by starting with arm exercises, increased by a few minutes each week. (He had to exercise infinite patience until he gained a perceptible amount of energy.)

With a nutrient-dense diet as well, he was soon able to stand for a few minutes by holding the back of a chair. After about a year of slow progress, he managed to take a few steps with a walker. Then he could manage them without a walker.

Eventually he was completely well, walking vigorously for several miles a day. His health was restored, and he has fought off the osteoporosis that would have made his bones fragile.

An experiment conducted by Dr. Herbert deVries, of the University of Southern California School of Medicine, dramatically demonstrates that it's never too late to take part in regular physical activity to gain fitness and ward off illness.

In *Solved: The Riddle of Illness*, Jim Scheer and I tell how Dr. deVries recruited men between the ages of 52 and 88 from Leisure World, a retirement colony at Laguna Hills, California. Some of them felt they were too old to exercise, but joined their friends anyhow.[7]

Put on a carefully monitored exercise routine daily—usually for no more than 15 minutes—participants showed surprising improvement: 35 percent greater breathing capacity and 30 percent increased ability of blood to transport oxygen to tissues. They also realized increased ability to relax and release pent-up feelings of frustration, aggression and hostility.

∾ 8 ∾

PIONEERING RESEARCH

Important research into osteoporosis, into the probabilities for developing this condition and new devices for measuring bone degeneration is being conducted by the University of California at San Francisco (UCSF), one of the world's leaders in such investigation.[1]

A new study by UCSF's Steven R. Cummings, professor of medicine, epidemiology and biostatistics, discloses that women with the highest risk of hip fractures are those who have lost weight since young adulthood, who have had a fracture of any kind after age 50 or those whose mother had had a hip fracture.

Raloxifene and Droloxifene, two new drugs, are being studied in several different trials on thousands of women volunteers to determine their effectiveness against osteoporosis. Like estrogen and progesterone, these drugs appear to increase bone density and reduce cholesterol levels. However, these are only preliminary results in a long-term study.

Still another approach is being followed in UCSF pioneering research, testing potassium bicarbonate, naturally found in fruits and vegetables, as a dietary supplement to neutralize excess acid created by diets rich in high-protein animal foods.

This acid depletes calcium in bone and causes demineralization, increasing the risk of spine and hip fractures, says senior researcher Anthony Sebastian, professor of medicine. Postmenopausal women given potassium bicarbonate reduced the amount of calcium lost in the urine and showed an increase in formation of new bone.

A NATURAL HORMONE APPROACH

A sensation has been created by the research of Nancy Lane, San Francisco General Hospital associate professor of medicine, into administration of parathyroid gland hormone, a naturally-occurring substance which regulates the amount of calcium in the blood in the same way the thermostat on an air conditioner regulates the degree of cooling air.

High dosage of this hormone was revealed to increase and even restore bone in rats which had lost 50 percent of their bone density. Dr. Lane and Claude Arnaud, a UCSF professor of medicine and physiology, are now collaborating on a clinical trial to determine results of use of this hormone in patients who have experienced bone loss due to taking corticosteroids, commonly prescribed for rheumatoid arthritis, asthma and other ailments.

TRI-DIMENSIONAL BONE-VIEWING

UCSF researchers pioneered development of Quantitative Computed Tomography (QCT), an adaptation of conventional CT, now widely used to provide sensitive images of the spine.

Dr. Christopher Cann, professor of radiology and bioengineering, has now extended QCT by using three-dimensional measurements and a mathematical model that he devised to estimate bone strength.

Dr. Cann's patented method can be used to predict who may be at risk to have bone fractures and are therefore candidates for preventive osteoporosis treatment. This diagnostic instrument can also be used to indicate to practitioners the best treatment to follow.

Another viewing device, quantitative ultrasound, can help doctors estimate the degree of hip fracture by viewing the heel bone and other parts of the limbs, states Harry Genant, professor of radiological medicine and orthopedic surgery.

Ultrasound devices have an advantage over many other viewing instruments in that they do not expose patients to radiation, are relatively low cost and, best of all, are portable.

Another giant step forward—this to examine how bone structures heal—is a system for three-dimensional high-resolution microscopy being used by UCSF's Nancy Lane and John Kinney, at the Lawrence Livermore National Laboratory.

Eventually, such devices will be available in most large hospitals and osteoporosis clinics to make diagnosis and effectiveness of treatment precisely measurable and treatable.

∞ 9 ∞

THE SUMMING UP

A popular song of another day recommended that we "accentuate the positive and *eee*liminate the negative." This surely applies to prevention and/or reversal of osteoporosis.

Let's start by eliminating the following negatives or at least minimizing them: heavy intake of alcohol, coffee, sugar, carbonated beverages, meat and eggs—all of which limit the amount of calcium being absorbed and retained.

Most soft drinks contain liberal amounts of phosphoric acid. Meat and egg yolks are rich in phosphorus. If the calcium-phosphorus ratio tilts in favor of phosphorus, phosphorus combines with calcium and strong-arms it out of the body, a process which can undermine bones and teeth.

Additionally, too high an intake of protein interferes with calcium absorption, as is noted by many

authorities. Although estimates of the daily requirement for protein vary, I follow a program similar to
that advocated by Richard A. Kunin, M.D., the au-
thor of *Mega-Nutrition* (p. 267): roughly one gram
of protein for every two pounds of body weight.
This adds up to 75 grams of protein for a person
weighing 150 pounds. How much is a gram? About
1/28 ounce.

A liberal intake of oxalic acid and phytic acid—
the former in beet greens, chard, rhubarb and spinach—and the latter in whole grains—also tends to
remove available calcium from the body.

Now let's deal with the positives: supplements and
regular physical exercise, starting with taking in
enough vitamin D: usually 400 I.U. daily, necessary
for calcium absorption and utilization.

It is not always possible to derive our vitamin D
from the interaction of the sun's rays with our skin.
In temperate or cold climates, the sun distances itself
too much from us in the fall and winter seasons to
be effective in this way. Also, in areas of frequent
cloudiness or persistent smog, the sun's beneficial
rays are intercepted and consequently diminished.

Remember that the amount of vitamin D added
to milk has been found to be unreliable. Best food
and supplement sources are cod liver oil, sardines,
salmon, tuna, egg yolk, mushroom, shrimp and sunflower seeds.

Additional calcium doesn't always stop or reverse
osteoporosis. However, in addition to foods rich in

calcium, I recommend that my patients take a capsule containing 1000 mg of calcium and 500 mg of magnesium. Some of them have had excellent results ingesting an additional 500 mg of magnesium, making for a one-to-one ratio.

Cow's milk is usually considered the best food source of calcium. However cheeses rate five to six times higher in calcium content, and milk-intolerant people can substitute a few ounces of cheese or a cup or two of yogurt for a glass of milk without the usual side effects.

Sesame seeds, sardines and canned salmon (the soft bones are in them), brewer's yeast, carob, soybeans, almonds and Brazil nuts and leafy green vegetables are excellent food and supplement sources of calcium.

Consider that researcher Morris Notelovitz, M.D. found that calcium supplements are most efficiently absorbed before bedtime when taken with a glass of milk. A cup of yogurt or several ounces of cheese or other calcium-rich foods can be substituted by milk intolerants. Calcium levels are low in the evening, and, at that time, there are not a lot of foods competing with calcium for absorption.

Foods richest in magnesium are kelp, blackstrap molasses, sunflower seeds, wheat germ, almonds, soybeans, Brazil nuts, pistachios and soy lecithin.

I recommend that patients take a 30 to 50 mg supplement of manganese daily. Best food bets for manganese are buckwheat, oats, hazelnuts, wheat, pecans, barley, Brazil nuts, sunflower seeds, peas, beans and walnuts.

Although only three mg of boron are needed daily, this amount usually can be obtained by eating several fruits and vegetables daily: apples, pears, peaches, leafy vegetables, peas and beans and nuts. However, for those who don't eat enough of these foods, several brands of boron supplements contain three mg in a tablet or capsule.

In addition to dietary factors important to preventing or recovering from osteoporosis is regular exercise—preferably weight-bearing. Like muscle, bone becomes stronger and more developed with use. One reason for osteoporosis is a decline in physical activity as people age.

Research by Everett L. Smith, Ph.D., authority on the biology of aging at the University of Wisconsin, Peter Jacobson, at the University of North Carolina (Chapel Hill) and R. Bruce Martin, M.D., director of Orthopedic Research at West Virginia Medical Center, demonstrates that any regular aerobic exercise protects or grows bones—fast and vigorous walking, jogging or running, tennis, aerobic dancing and even gardening.

Of course, it is necessary to get your doctor's approval before launching an ambitious exercise program, because small, thin and fragile bones could possibly collapse.

The hormonal approach brings mixed blessings. Estrogen, in most instances, stops bone loss, but it adds none. However, in some studies it even permits a slight bone loss. Further, it may cause breast and uterine cancer and generate other side effects—abnormal blood clotting which could contribute to strokes or heart attacks, breast tenderness, jaundice, nausea, sleeplessness and depression.

As pointed out by Alan R. Gaby, M.D., the hormone estriol can accomplish what estrogen does, but with fewer side effects and hazards. It is the "forgotten estrogen." However, proper nutrition and exercise prove to be more effective in preventing and reversing bone loss than estrogen or estriol. So one can recommend the hormonal modality only with reservations.

A task force method brings best results in stopping and then reversing osteoporosis—eliminating the negative, enhancing the diet with real foods and supplements, and, of course, performing regular vigorous forms of exercise. Trying to reverse osteoporosis without daily physical activity is like attempting to lose weight without vigorous aerobic exercise.

The task force approach has worked for my patients. So I know that it is valid and helpful. It is the best method I know for coping with osteoporosis, an insidious, undermining, life-shortening degenerative disease.

❧ REFERENCES ❧

Chapter 1
THE ENEMY WORKS UNDERCOVER

❧ REFERENCES ❧

Chapter 1
THE ENEMY WORKS UNDERCOVER

1. "Bone Loss Linked to Early Menstruation Halt," *Register* (Orange County, Cal.), February 3, 1984, Section B, p. 10.
2. Ibid.
3. "Bone Disease Found to Strike the Young, Too," Associated Press release, September 14, 1983.
4. "Jawbone Shrinkage: A Symptom of Osteoporosis," *The Encyclopedia of Common Disease.* Emmaus, Pa.: Rodale Press, Inc., 1982, pp. 1181–1182.
5. "Gray Hair and Osteoporosis," *NNFA Today*, December 1994, p. 5.
6. Donald, Alan, "Coping with Osteoporosis," *Bestways*, November 1986, pp. 14–24.

Chapter 2
Junky Foods, Junky Bones

1. Hendler, Sheldon Saul, M.D., Ph.D., *The Purification Prescription*. New York: William Morrow and Company, Inc., 1991, p. 44.
2. Garrison, Robert Jr., M.A., R.Ph. and Somer, Elizabeth, M.A., R.D., *The Nutrition Desk Reference*. New Canaan, Conn.: Keats Publishing, Inc., 1995, p. 160.
3. Gaby, Alan R., M.D., *Preventing and Reversing Osteoporosis*. Rocklin, Cal.: Prima Publishing, 1994, pp. 14–15.
4. *Practical Encyclopedia of Natural Healing*. Emmaus, Pa.: Rodale Press, Inc., 1983, p. 70.
5. *Preventing and Reversing Osteoporosis*, p. 13.
6. Ibid.
7. "Boning Up on Osteoporosis," *Science News*, August 27, 1983, p. 140.
8. Murray, Frank, *The Big Family Guide to All the Minerals*. New Canaan, Conn.: Keats Publishing, Inc., 1995, pp. 99–100.
9. Ibid.
10. *The Nutrition Desk Reference*, p. 152.
11. Brown, Susan E., Ph.D., *Better Bones, Better Body*. New Canaan, Conn.: Keats Publishing, Inc., 1996, p. 128.
12. *The Big Family Guide to All the Minerals*. p. 96.
13. Long, Ruth Yale, Ph.D., *Home Study Course in the New Nutrition*. New Canaan, Conn.: Keats Publishing, Inc., 1989, Lesson 7–3.
14. Ibid.
15. Ibid.
16. *The Nutrition Desk Reference*, p. 241.
17. *Preventing and Reversing Osteoporosis*, p. 185.

18. Ibid., p. 187.
19. *Home Study Course in the New Nutrition,* Lesson 8–5.

Chapter 3
GET OUT IN THE SUN!

1. Lillyquist, Michael J., *Sunlight and Health.* New York: Dodd, Mead and Company, 1985, p. 8.
2. Ibid., p. 15.
3. Newbold, H.L., M.D., *Mega-Nutrients.* Los Angeles: The Body Press, 1987, p. 274.
4. Donald, Alan, "Coping with Osteoporosis," *Bestways,* November 1986, p. 16–46.
5. *Sunlight and Health,* p. 21.
6. Ibid., p. 65.
7. Ibid., pp. 23, 24.
8. *Mega-Nutrients,* p. 275.
9. Ibid., p. 280.
10. Ibid., pp. 280–281.
11. Ibid., p. 276.

Chapter 4
BEAT OSTEOPOROSIS WITH SUPERNUTRITION

1. Salaman, Maureen and Scheer, James F., *Foods That Heal,* Statford Press, Menlo Park, CA.: 1989, pp. 386–387.
2. Ibid.
3. Izawa, I., et al., *Calcification Tissue International,* 36 (1981): 623–30.
4. Meshawari, U.R., et al., *American Journal of Clinical Nutrition* 36 (2) (1982): 211–18.
5. "Early Prevention of Osteoporosis," *Los Angeles Times,* June 25, 1986, Part 2, p. 1.
6. Ibid.

7. "Bone Disease may Cripple Older Women," *Los Angeles Times,* August 19, 1983, Part 2, p. 1.
8. Lipski, M.S., *Digestive Wellness.* New Canaan, Conn.: Keats Publishing, Inc., 1996, p. 200.
9. Rogers, Sherry A., M.D., "Calcium: the Killer," *Organica News,* Winter 1990, p. 19.
10. Langer, Stephen, M.D. and Scheer, James F., *Beat Osteoporosis for Life.* New York: Instant Improvement, 1989, pp. 7–8.
11. "Nutrients and Bone Health," a publication of the Wright-Gaby Institute, August 1988, p. 1.
12. *The Complete Book of Vitamins.* Emmaus, Pa.: Rodale Press, Inc., 1977, p. 136.
13. "Nutrients and Bone Health," p. 3.
14. Ibid.
15. Ibid.
16. Ibid.
17. Ibid.
18. Ibid.
19. Ibid.
20. *Sunlight and Health,* p. 70.
21. Gallop, P.M., et al., "Carboxylated Calcium-Binding Protein and Vitamin K," *New England Journal of Medicine,* 1980; 60: 1268–1269.
22. Ibid.
23. *Beat Osteoporosis for Life,* p. 10.
24. Robert, D., et al., "Hypercalciuria During Experimental Vitamin K Deficiency in the Rat," *Calcification Tissue International,* 1986; 37: 143–147.
25. Ibid.
26. Cohen, L., Kitzes, R., "Infrared Spectroscopy and Magnesium Content of Bone Material in Osteoporotic Women," *Israel Journal of Medical Science,* 1981; 17: 1123–1125.

27. Landy, Liz, "Gallup Survey Finds Majority of American Diets Lack Sufficient Magnesium—at Potential Cost to Health," *Searle News,* September 21, 1994.
28. Amdur, M.O., et al., "The Need for Manganese in Bone Development of the Rat," *Proceedings of the Society of Experimental Biological Medicine,* 1945; 59: 254–255.
29. Raloff, Janet, "Reasons for Boning Up on Manganese," *Science News,* 1986, September 27, p. 199.
30. "Nutrients and Bone Health," p. 3.
31. Ibid.
32. Ibid.
33. *The Big Family Guide to All the Minerals,* p. 347.
34. "Nutrients and Bone Health," p. 3.
35. Langer, Stephen, M.D. and Scheer, James F., *How to Win at Weight Loss,* Rochester, Vt.: Thorsons Publishers, 1987, p. 66.
36. Atik, O.S., "Zinc and Senile Osteoporosis," *Journal of the American Geriatric Society,* 1983; 31: 790–791.

Chapter 5
GET MORE MILEAGE OUT OF YOUR CALCIUM

1. Scheer, James F., "Osteoporosis: More Than a Calcium Deficiency," *Health Freedom News,* June/July, 1990, pp. 9–14.
2. "Calcium: Beneficial to Bones and More," *The Healthy Cell News,* Spring/Summer, 1995, p. 17.
3. "Calcium: The Killer," p. 19.
4. Gaby, Alan R., M.D., "Non-Dairy Sources of Calcium," *Townsend Letter for Doctors,* July, 1990, p. 430.
5. Personal Communication with Morris Notelovitz, M.D., University of Florida, June 1990.

6. Hoffer, Abram, M.D., *Orthomolecular Medicine for Physicians*. New Canaan, Conn.: Keats Publishing, Inc., 1989, pp. 84–85.

7. Zeitlin-Kravets, Barbara, "Calcium Goes Beyond Bones," *Health Freedom News*, October 1986, p. 16.

Chapter 6
THE ESTROGEN DILEMMA

1. Vils, Ursula, "Rx Warning on Dangers of Estrogen," *Los Angeles Times*, January 22, 1976, Part 1, pp. 1–7.

2. "Boning Up on Osteoporosis," *Science News*, July 27, 1983, p. 141.

3. Ibid.

4. "Two Studies Reach Opposite Findings on Estrogen," *Los Angeles Times*, October 24, 1985, Part 2, p. 1.

5. *Preventing and Reversing Osteoporosis*, pp. 131–132.

6. "Treating Post-Menopausal Bone Loss," *Los Angeles Times*, Part 7, pp. 20–21.

7. Ibid.

8. Ibid.

9. *Preventing and Reversing Osteoporosis*, p. 127.

10. Reitz, Rosetta, *Menopause: A Positive Approach*, New York: Chilton Book Company, 1989, p. 56.

11. Mindell, Earl, R.Ph., Ph.D., *What You Should Know About Natural Health for Women*. New Canaan, Conn.: Keats Publishing, Inc., 1996, p. 65.

12. Lindsay, Robert, M.D., "Osteoporosis Update: Strategies to Counteract Bone Loss, Prevent Fracture," *Consultant*, July 1996, pp. 1387–1395.

13. Prior, Jerilynn C., "Progesterone and the Prevention of Osteoporosis," *The Canadian Journal of Ob/Gyn & Women's Health Care* 3.4 (1991): 178–184.

14. *Preventing and Reversing Osteoporosis,* pp. 150–154.
15. "Osteoporosis Update: Strategies to Counteract Bone Loss, Prevent Fracture." pp. 1387–1395.
16. Riggs, B.L., "A New Option for Treating Osteoporosis," *New England Journal of Medicine,* 323: 124–125, 1990.
17. "Osteoporosis Update: Strategies to Counteract Bone Loss, Prevent Fracture."

Chapter 7
SOLVED: THE RIDDLE OF ILLNESS

1. "Boning Up on Osteoporosis," p. 140.
2. Ibid.
3. "Bone Disease May Cripple Older Women," *Los Angeles Times,* August 18, 1983, Part 2, p. 1.
4. Scheer, James F., "Osteoporosis: More Than A Calcium Deficiency," *Health Freedom News,* June/July, 1990, p. 9.
5. *Preventing and Reversing Osteoporosis,* p. 222.
6. Lloyd, Tom, Ph.D., et al., "Calcium Supplementation and Bone Mineral Density in Adolescent Girls," *Journal of the American Medical Association,* August 18, 1993, Vol. 270, No. 7, pp. 841–843.
7. Langer, Stephen, M.D. and Scheer, James F., *Solved: The Riddle of Illness,* Second Edition. New Canaan, Conn.: Keats Publishing, Inc., 1995, p. 176.

Chapter 8
PIONEERIING RESEARCH

1. Higbee, Rebecca, "UCSF's Key Players in Osteoporosis Research," *UCSF Newsbreak,* Vol. II, #11, June 1, 1995.

INDEX

Index

STEPHEN E. LANGER, M.D. practices preventive medicine in Berkeley, California. He specializes in anti-aging and in the treatment of chronic fatigue, and is available for consultation at (510) 548-7384.